Behavioral Science/Psychiatry:
Review for New National Boards

Behavioral Science/Psychiatry:
Review for New National Boards

Julia B. Frank, M.D.
Associate Professor
       and
Nadia Krupnikova, M.D.
Clinical Assistant Professor
Department of Psychiatry and Behavioral Sciences
The George Washington University Medical Center
Washington, D.C.

J&S

J&S Publishing Company Inc., Alexandria, Virginia

J&S

Composition and Layout: Ronald C. Bohn, Ph. D.
Cover Design: Kurt E. Johnson, Ph. D.
Printing Supervisor: Robert Perotti, Jr.
Printing: Goodway Graphics, Springfield, Virginia

Library of Congress Catalog Card Number 97-070532

ISBN 1-888308-00-1

© 1998 by J & S Publishing Company, Inc., Alexandria, Virginia

10 9 8 7 6 5 4 3 2 1

Dedication

Julia B. Frank, M.D. would like to add the following dedication.

Choose the BEST response

As the daughter of a prominent academic psychiatrist and a trained psychotherapist, I can truly say I learned psychiatry at my parent's knee. As the mother of three lively and magnificently complex children, I apply behavioral science every waking moment of every day. Were it not for the many sacrifices and unstinting support of my husband, I could not also practice psychiatry in an academic setting where I continue to learn and grow. In light of these incalculable debts, this book is lovingly dedicated to

(A) Jerome and Elizabeth Frank
(B) Naomi, Abigail and Rebecca Graber
(C) Mark A. Graber
(D) All of the above

The answer is self-evident.

Table of Contents

Preface

This book is designed to prepare medical students in just 1-2 days for the behavioral science and psychiatry sections of the USMLE, Steps 1 and 2. Such condensed review is possible because the exam no longer rewards an encyclopedic knowledge of the basic sciences. Instead, the new exams test knowledge of the scientific basis of disease and the ability to apply basic scientific information in clinical reasoning. The most efficient way to study for the new exam is 1) to review only the most relevant material from each basic science course and 2) to focus on the application of this information to the solution of clinical problems. This book exemplifies such a streamlined approach.

Because all material conforms to the **Diagnostic and Statistical Manual-IV** of the American Psychiatric Association, published in 1994, advanced students and even residents may use this text to revise and update psychiatric knowledge based on earlier classifcatory schemes. First and second year students may also find our items provide a useful self-test of the material they study in behavioral science and introduction to psychiatry courses. Taking an hour to answer the relevant sections during the week when a topic is presented in lecture will help students evaluate their grasp of the material. Detailed self-knowledge will allow the student to focus on the topics that need the most attention.

This book supplements but cannot substitute for one of the many excellent general psychiatry textbooks available, three of which comprise our major primary sources:

Kaplan, HI, Sadock, BJ and Grebb, JA. *Kaplan and Saddock's Synopsis of Psychiatry*, 7th ed, 1994.
Andreasen, NE and Black, DW. *Introductory Textbook of Psychiatry*, 2nd ed, 1995.
Stoudemire, A. *Clinical Psychiatry for Medical Students*, 2nd ed, 1994.

The advantage of such books is comprehensiveness. Their main flaw is the tendency to give equal weight to every point. In psychiatry in particular, the desire to be scientific and evenhanded sometimes prompts authors of textbooks to finesse areas of continuing disagreement and to gloss over the distinction between facts, hypotheses, theories, and wild speculations. The single-best-choice format and clinical focus of this book, by contrast, require the authors and the reader to weigh information critically, subjecting it to the acid test of clinical usefulness.

The student who answers every item and reads all the tutorials in this book can cover the most relevant information from behavioral science and introduction to psychiatry courses in just 2 days. Many facts are presented in the context of a vignette drawn from the authors' extensive clinical experience. We hope this emphasis on clinical application will enhance your understanding and recall of information. Even before the first clinical rotation, we want you to see how knowledgeable physicians use behavioral science information to understand the course of clinical disease and the significance of abnormal findings. With the wind of this book at your back, we hope you sail through the wards as well as the boards.

Julia B. Frank, M.D.
Nadia Krupnikova, M.D.
Washington, DC
January, 1998

Acknowledgements

The authors would like to thank Kurt E. Johnson, Ph. D., President and Publisher, J & S Publishing Company, Inc. for the opportunity to write this book, for his expert advice, flexibility, and encouragement throughout the project; and, Ronald C. Bohn, Ph. D., Associate Professor, Department of Anatomy, The George Washington University Medical Center for his assistance in formatting the final documents for publication.

Disclaimer

The clinical information presented in this book is accurate for the purposes of review for licensure examinations but in no way should be used to treat patients or substituted for modern clinical training. Proper diagnosis and treatment of patients requires comprehensive evaluation of all symptoms, careful monitoring for adverse responses to treatment and assessment of the long-term consequences of therapeutic intervention.

Figure Credits

Figures 1.1 and 1.2 From Kendall, R.E. and Zeally, A.K. Companion to Psychiatric Studies, ed. 3, ©1985 reprinted with permission of Churchill-Livingston, New York.

Figure 6.1 From Stoudemire, A., M.D., ed. Clinical Psychiatry for Medical Students, ed. 2, ©1994 reprinted with permission of J.B. Lippincott, Philadelphia.

Figure 10.1 and 10.2 From Psychiatric Annals, 17: 437-445, ©1987 reprinted with permission of Slack Inc., Thorofare, N.J.

CHAPTER I
NEUROBIOLOGY IN PSYCHIATRY

Items 1-4

Figure 1.1 is a labelled diagram of medial brain structures.

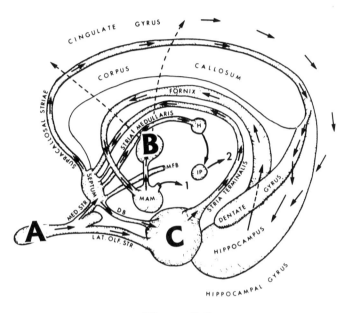

Figure 1.1

1. Structure A is the

   (A) amygdala
   (B) hypothalamus
   (C) olfactory bulb
   (D) anterior nucleus of the thalamus
   (E) pons

2. Structure B is the

   (A) anterior nucleus of the thalamus
   (B) hypothalamus
   (C) amygdala
   (D) raphe nucleus
   (E) cerebellum

3.   Structure C is the

      (A)   stria terminalis
      (B)   amygdala
      (C)   parahippocampal area
      (D)   arcuate nucleus
      (E)   substantia nigra

4.   The structures identified above are linked together in a functional brain circuit called the

      (A)   limbic system
      (B)   reticular activating system
      (C)   subcortical thalamic projections
      (D)   rhinencephalon
      (E)   brainstem

ANSWERS AND TUTORIAL ON ITEMS 1-4

The answers are: **1-C; 2-A; 3-B; 4-A**. **Figure 1.2** shows a fully labeled picture of medial structures in the brain.

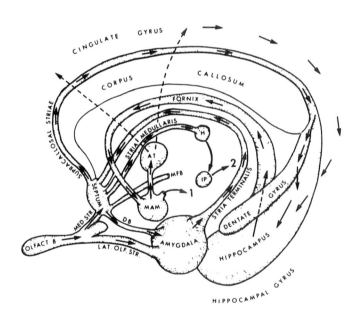

Figure 1.2

The **limbic system** or Papez circuit is a network of brain centers located in and around the medial temporal lobes. Its main structures include the olfactory bulb, the hypothalamus, amygdala, mammillary bodies, anterior nucleus of thalamus, hippocampus, parahippocampal area, and septal nuclei. Connecting pathways include the fimbria, the stria terminalis, the medial forebrain bundle, the striatum, the septum, and the anterior commissure. While these areas project to and receive inputs from many areas of the neocortex, their rich interconnections can function more or less autonomously, leading to emotions and behavior not fully represented in or modified by conscious thought.

Functioning of the limbic system subserves many of the **primary motivations of human behavior**. These functions include memory, aggression, sexual desire and response, exploratory behavior, anxiety, attention, pleasure, activity level, and feeding. The limbic system also has rich connections to the locus ceruleus and the raphe nucleus, the major norepinephrine- and serotonin-containing centers of the brain. These, in concert with the reticular activating system, regulate arousal, sleep-wake cycles and sensory perception.

Items 5-9

Matching. Choose the **BEST** match between the brain area in the answers and the description of its functional role in the items below. Answers may be used once, more than once, or not at all.

(A)   Amygdala
(B)   Broca's area
(C)   Hippocampus
(D)   Hypothalamus
(E)   Thalamus
(F)   Pons
(G)   Motor cortex
(H)   Sensory cortex
(I)   Locus ceruleus
(J)   Temporal association areas
(K)   Median raphe nucleus

5.   Area of the medial temporal lobe which, if damaged bilaterally, leads to loss of short-term memory and capacity for new learning.

6.   Center of serotonin-containing cell bodies in the brain, implicated in regulation of sleep-wake cycles.

7.   Center of adrenergic cell bodies in the upper brainstem. Thought to be an important target area for many antipanic and antidepressant drugs.

8.   Temporal lobe area which, if damaged bilaterally along with overlying portions of surrounding cortex, produces docility, compulsive oral activity, indiscriminate sexual activity, and loss of fear (Klüver-Bucy's syndrome). Stimulation of this structure produces apparent rage in animals.

9.   Large brain center which receives sensory inputs in every modality except smell and relays this to specific areas of the neocortex. Similarly relays cortical messages to somatic and visceral effector neurons. The posterior portion of this area is particularly important for relaying pain messages to and from the cortex.

ANSWERS AND TUTORIAL ON ITEMS 5-9

The answers are: **5-C; 6-K; 7-I; 8-A; 9-E**. Stimulation or controlled lesioning of the **limbic system** in animals and the study of humans with epileptic foci, tumors, or injuries in this area provide clues to the clinical relevance of limbic functions. In general, destructive lesions must be bilateral to cause clear behavioral changes. Bilateral destruction of the **hippocampus** leads to loss of short-term memory and the capacity for new learning.

Both the limbic system and the cortex receive regulatory inputs from nuclei in the **brainstem**, with reciprocal fibers modulating the activity of these cells. Two nuclei of great relevance to psychiatry are the **median raphe nucleus**, center for **serotonin**-containing **cell bodies**, and the **locus ceruleus**, where **adrenergic cell bodies** cluster in large numbers. Brainstem nuclei regulate the **vegetative state** of the organism: level of arousal, sleep-wake cycles, breathing, heart rate, temperature, and so on. The reciprocal direct and mediated pathways between these centers and the cortex underlie the complex interactions between humans' conscious beliefs, moods, and interpretations of the world and their biological functioning.

Stimulation of the **amygdalae** or the midbrain gray matter causes apparent **rage** reactions in laboratory animals, as does lesioning of the septum. Stimulation of other parts of the amygdala in laboratory animals and surgical patients produces **fear**. Humans with epileptic foci in these areas may experience irritability, rage or painful anxiety and arousal during and following seizures. In monkeys, bilateral lesions of the amygdalae and surrounding mantle of hippocampal cells produce the **Klüver-Bucy's syndrome**: compulsive oral activity, docility, decreased ability to identify familiar objects, lack of anxiety, and indiscriminate sexual activity. The same lesion in humans leads to apathy, bulimia, and hypersexuality.

The **thalamus**, whose anterior nuclei are part of the limbic system, is the major way station in which peripheral sensory information is received, organized and transmitted via thalamocortical tracts to specific cortical areas. Responses are then conveyed back to the thalamus via corticothalamic tracts. These originate in many areas including the frontal cortex, precentral and postcentral gyri, Heschl's gyri, the posterior parietal region and adjacent areas of the temporal lobe. These fibers synapse in the thalamus, from which efferent spinothalamic tracts pass to synapse on both peripheral motor neurons and the neurons of the autonomic nervous system.

A 16-year-old boy is brought to the doctor after apparently trying to take off his clothes during the showing of a filmstrip. He describes having started to see wavy lines on the screen, then experiencing a brief period of mental blankness, followed by fatigue and headache.

10.   The **MOST** probable diagnosis of this patient is

    (A)   grand mal epilepsy
    (B)   migraine behavioral syndrome
    (C)   partial complex seizure
    (D)   exhibitionism
    (E)   schizophreniform disorder

11.   The patient and his family should be questioned about

    (A)   history of irritability or violence
    (B)   history of sexual molestation
    (C)   experiences of *déjà vu, jamais vu,* depersonalization and inexplicable emotional states
    (D)   A and C only
    (E)   A, B, and C

12.   Diagnostic evaluation should involve

    (A)   MRI or CT scan
    (B)   clinical neurological examination
    (C)   sleep-deprived EEG
    (D)   projective tests. e.g., the Rorschach or Thematic Apperception Test
    (E)   A, B and C only

13.   Treatment should include

    (A)   carbamazepine or valproic acid
    (B)   behavior therapy to reduce compulsions
    (C)   lithium carbonate to reduce impulsivity
    (D)   ergotamine

14.   After ten to twenty years, this patient is at risk to develop

    (A)   dementia
    (B)   antisocial personality disorder
    (C)   chronic psychosis resembling schizophrenia
    (D)   bulimia nervosa
    (E)   pain disorder

ANSWERS AND TUTORIAL ON ITEMS 10-14

The answers are: **10-C; 11-D; 12-E; 13-A; 14-C**. This set of items pertains to neuropsychiatric syndromes linked to limbic system dysfunction. Because the electroencephalogram (EEG) measures only the top few millimeters of brain electrical activity, epileptic foci deep in the limbic system are difficult to detect. When they fire without spreading to the rest of the brain, they may produce symptoms and behaviors that are easily mistaken for primary psychiatric disorders. Seizures confined to limbic structures are called **partial complex seizures** (formerly temporal lobe epilepsy). Recognized aspects of partial complex seizures include preseizure auras involving sensory distortions (olfactory and gustatory hallucinations, visual distortions; rarely, abdominal pain). During the ictal phase, patients may show stereotypic, elemental motor activity (standing and sitting, buttoning and unbuttoning), and disruptions of cognitive functioning (trance, depersonalization, repetitive thoughts). A partial seizure may also generalize to the rest of the brain, producing a grand mal seizure. Patients are typically amnestic for the ictal phase of either a grand mal or partial seizure and sometimes for events immediately beforehand (**anterograde amnesia**). Intense dysphoria, anxiety or rage may occur in conjunction with partial seizures and also in periods far removed from the actual seizure.

Organized, directed, violent behavior rarely if ever occurs during a seizure. However, violent behavior may occur interictally in patients with partial complex seizures or those with nonepileptic EEG abnormalities in the temporal lobes. Interictal irritability is very common. Frequent *déjà vu* or *jamais vu* and feelings of depersonalization are other interictal clues that a patient may have partial complex seizures. Over many years, patients with partial complex seizures may develop personality changes, including passivity, unusual sexual behavior, loss of sexual interest, obsessiveness, religious preoccupations and even a chronic psychosis that closely resembles chronic schizophrenia. In patients with grand mal epilepsy, these changes are found more commonly in those with primary lesions in the limbic system than in those with other foci.

The diagnosis of partial complex seizures is sometimes hard to confirm. EEG abnormalities are most easily detected during the transition from waking to sleep, so it is best to perform the EEG on sleep-deprived patients who fall asleep while being recorded. While partial complex seizures may be idiopathic, a clinical neurologic examination and brain imaging studies may detect structural lesions that account for the abnormal electrical activity. Projective psychological tests, though often helpful in studying personality and uncovering psychosis, have little place in the evaluation of neurological disorders, even those with psychological symptoms. Neuropsychological tests would be of greater value.

Complex partial seizures respond best to **anticonvulsants**, with carbamazepine and valproic acid often more effective and less toxic than phenytoin, barbiturates or benzodiazepines. Lithium, which may reduce impulsiveness and violence, is **analeptic** (lowers the seizure threshold), and not advisable as a single agent in patients with seizures. Behavior therapy is sometimes effective for compulsions, but not for those related to epilepsy. **Ergotamine** is used specifically for the treatment of migraine headaches.

Items 15-17

A 55-year-old man with a history of heavy alcohol use comes to the emergency room for treatment of an infected gash in his hand. He is not currently intoxicated. His clothes fit loosely, and he mentions that he thinks he has lost weight since becoming homeless "sometime this year." In preparation for giving him antibiotics, he gets an intravenous infusion of 5% dextrose solution. Two hours later, he is confused, agitated, and ataxic, with bilateral sixth nerve palsies (intranuclear ophthalmoplegia) and nystagmus.

15.   This patient is **MOST** likely exhibiting

    (A)   alcoholic ketoacidosis
    (B)   Wernicke's encephalopathy
    (C)   Friedreich's ataxia
    (D)   sepsis
    (E)   malnutrition

16.   Immediate treatment should include

    (A)   100 mg of thiamine in each bag of IV fluid
    (B)   insulin, glucose, potassium and saline
    (C)   vitamin B_{12} IM and oral folic acid for three days
    (D)   intravenous lorazepam 2 mg every four hours until agitation subsides

17.   The patient is treated and admitted to the hospital. In three days, his wound is healing, and he no longer shows signs of neuropathy. However, his mental status is remarkable for mild confusion, even though he seems awake and alert. He is socially appropriate and denies hallucinations, delusions or ideas of reference. He is oriented to place but not date, able to give his correct date of birth, do simple calculations, and provide the correct address of the house where he lived for 10 years. However, he cannot recall even one of three objects at five minutes. He seems unable to remember what he ate at his most recent meal. When asked by the examiner if he remembers the two of them having met and enjoyed an evening together, he cheerfully says he does, though in fact this never occurred. Vital signs are BP 110/60; P 82 and regular. Liver function tests, serum electrolytes and BUN/creatinine are all within normal limits, except for slight elevation of alkaline phosphatase to 652 u/ml (upper limit of normal=600 u/ml) and SGPT to 50 u/ml (upper limit of normal=35). CBC shows a hemoglobin of 11.3 gm/100 ml (nl 12-15 gm/ml); HCT of 37% (nl 40-50%); MCV of 101 fL (nl = 82-92)

Having recovered from his presenting illness, this patient is now exhibiting

    (A)   malingering
    (B)   multi-infarct dementia
    (C)   alcohol amnestic syndrome (Korsakoff's syndrome)
    (D)   Wernicke's encephalopathy

ANSWERS AND TUTORIAL ON ITEMS 15-17

The answers are: **15-B; 16-A; 17-C**. Ablation or destruction of limbic areas highlights the role of **limbic areas** in the processing and storage of **memory**. Because of the protection afforded by the redundancy of having two hemispheres with overlapping functions, tumors, injuries or infarctions affecting limbic areas are often silent, unless they cause pressure effects or electrical excitation. Toxic or metabolic damage, which typically affects symmetrical areas, can, by contrast, have dramatic impact. The most common, clinically significant example is that of **thiamine deficiency**, which occurs in malnutrition, especially among alcoholics.

Acute thiamine deficiency produces **Wernicke's encephalopathy**. The cardinal features of this condition are delirium with ataxia, oculomotor dysfunction (especially 6th nerve palsy-intranuclear ophthalmoplegia) and sometimes anisocoria.

Administering glucose to someone on the verge of thiamine deficiency can precipitate acute encephalopathy, because thiamine is a cofactor for the cerebral metabolism of glucose. Wernicke's encephalopathy is prevented or rapidly reversed by the administration of thiamine.

Chronic thiamine deficiency causes **alcohol-induced persisting amnestic disorder** (Korsakoff's syndrome). The main sites of damage are paraventricular, symmetrical lesions in the mammillary bodies, the thalamus, and the hypothalamus. Lesions may also occur in the midbrain, pons, medulla, fornix and cerebellum. Cerebellar and ocular signs may not be present. Diagnosis depends on a careful mental status examination. Patients with the alcohol amnestic syndrome have relatively preserved long-term memory, are socially appropriate, use language normally and can do simple calculations. Their profound recent memory loss seems so disproportionate to the rest of their mental status that observers may misdiagnose malingering--that is, willfully faking abnormality for some personal gain. Patients with the amnestic syndrome will occasionally try to conceal their deficits by confabulation, making up or agreeing to untrue scenarios given by the examiner. This is not the same thing as lying, but is often mistaken for it. The presence of mild macrocytosis and elevated liver enzymes is a common incidental finding in chronic alcoholics and does not explain the behavioral changes described.

Items 18-27

Choose the **BEST** response.

18.   The prefrontal cortex

    (A)   is much larger and more highly developed in humans than in other animals

    (B)   is defined as that part of the association cortex that receives projections from the medial dorsal nucleus of the thalamus

    (C)   has multiple reciprocal connections with the rest of the neocortex (somatic, visual, and auditory), the hippocampus and amygdala, and other thalamic nuclei

    (D)   A and C only

    (E)   A, B, and C

19. The anatomy and neurotransmitter regulation of the prefrontal cortex, combined with studies of injury to this area, suggest that its functions include all of the following **EXCEPT**:

   (A) temporal sequencing, planning
   (B) abstract thought/creative problem solving
   (C) attention, concentration
   (D) voluntary motor behavior
   (E) receptive and expressive language

Items 20-23

Damage to different areas of the cortex is associated with identifiable psychobehavioral syndromes. Match the **MOST** likely area of damage in the list of answers below with the description of clinical symptoms in the items below.

   (A) Superior temporal gyrus (Brodmann's area 22)
   (B) Orbital, medial prefrontal cortex (magnocellular projections of the medial dorsal thalamus)
   (C) Dorsolateral prefrontal cortex (parvicellular projections of the medial dorsal thalamus)
   (D) Dominant parietal lobe
   (E) Superior and inferior occipital gyri

20. Hyperkinesis, euphoria, loss of social judgment (inappropriate behavior), shallow emotional expression, childish humor with punning and word play (*witzelsucht*).

21. Loss of ability to comprehend spoken language, fluent aphasia.

22. Apathy, hypokinesis, inattentiveness, impoverished affect, paucity of speech, loss of abstract capacity.

23. Right/left disorientation, inability to write (agraphia) or calculate (acalculia), inability to localize fingers (finger agnosia).

Choose the **BEST** response.

24. Identify the **TRUE** statements about the relevance of brain function to psychiatric symptoms.

   (A) Delusions and hallucinations may be related to abnormal excitability in brain pathways related to memory.
   (B) The overproductive, disorganized speech seen in mania resembles fluent aphasia but with intact comprehension.
   (C) Left hemisphere strokes are more likely to result in depression than those on the right, suggesting that the left hemisphere normally modulates dysphoric emotions originating in the right hemisphere.
   (D) A and C only
   (E) A, B, and C

25. Positron emission tomography (PET) studies of people with obsessive-compulsive disorder have found

   (A) hypofunctioning of the prefrontal cortex
   (B) hyperfunctioning of the prefrontal cortex
   (C) hyperconnectivity of temporal association cortex
   (D) hyperfunctioning of septal nuclei
   (E) None of the above

26. A 43-year-old man with a history of schizophrenia no longer reports hallucinations or delusions. However, he spends many hours doing nothing, has trouble reading a book or watching a movie, and rarely speaks spontaneously or fluently. His grooming is poor and he is socially withdrawn. A PET scan is **MOST** likely to show

   (A) symmetrically decreased size of cerebral ventricles
   (B) decreased metabolic activity in the temporal lobes, increased occipital lobe activity
   (C) hypoactivity of the prefrontal lobes, enlarged cerebral ventricles
   (D) hyperactivity of the prefrontal lobes
   (E) None of the above

27. He is likely to have difficulty in performing on

   (A) the Wisconsin Card-Sorting Test
   (B) the Porteus Maze Test
   (C) Continuous Performance Testing
   (D) A and C only
   (E) A, B, and C

ANSWERS AND TUTORIAL ON ITEMS 18-27

The answers are: **18-E; 19-E; 20-B; 21-A; 22-C; 23-D; 24-E; 25-B; 26-C; 27-E**. Major psychiatric syndromes like **schizophrenia, mania** and **depression** all involve impairments in sensory processing, purposeful or volitional behavior, adaptation to the environment, and the regulation of strong emotion. All of these functions are affected by the functioning of the **prefrontal cortex**, an anatomic area bounded by the arcuate sulcus, the inferior precentral sulcus, and the anterior cingulate gyrus. These boundaries correspond to the cortical projections of the medial dorsal nucleus of the thalamus. The prefrontal cortex occupies 29% of the human cortex, compared to 17% of the cortex of chimpanzees.

The prefrontal cortex has widespread, reciprocal connections with the rest of the neocortex and the limbic system, as well as unidirectional projections to the basal ganglia. This dense network subserves a variety of important functions, including planning, temporal sequencing, abstract thought, problem solving, motility, attention, and the modulation of emotion. Lesions of these pathways impair "the capacity to pursue goal directed behavior based on the integration of environmental and internal cues." (Andreasen, NC and Black, DW, *Introductory Textbook of Psychiatry*, 2nd ed., Washington, DC: APA Press, 1995, p. 135.)

Receptive and expressive language are somewhat localized in **Broca's area** (posterior frontal cortex) and **Wernicke's area** (superior temporal gyrus).

Damage to the **medial-orbital portions of the prefrontal cortex**, which correspond to the magnocellular projections of the medial dorsal thalamus, is followed by euphoria, shallow emotions, disinhibition of sexual and aggressive impulses, peculiar verbal humor and distractibility. This syndrome occurred in patients who underwent **prefrontal lobotomy** for severe depression or psychosis in the 1940s and 1950s.

Wernicke's area in the superior temporal gyrus (auditory association cortex) is the site of damage in patients with fluent aphasia. These patients are unable to comprehend spoken language and produce fluent, disorganized speech. Patients with **mania** also have fluent, disorganized speech, although their auditory comprehension is intact.

Posterior lesions of the prefrontal cortex, corresponding to the parvicellular projections of the medial dorsal thalamus, produce apathy, poverty of speech, hypokinesis, decreased drive or initiative, and diminished capacity to abstract. This syndrome resembles the deficit state of **schizophrenia**.

Damage to the **dominant parietal lobe** (visual, tactile and auditory association areas) leads to **Gerstmann's syndrome**: agraphia, acalculia (loss of previously acquired abilities to write and calculate), right-left disorientation, and finger agnosia (inability to localize fingers).

Damage to the **superior or inferior occipital gyri** leads to various problems of **visual recognition**, including cortical blindness, prosopagnosia (inability to recognize faces), color agnosia, and alexia (inability to read).

Various psychiatric disorders are known or hypothesized to involve dysfunction of various brain areas. **Delusions and hallucinations** may involve the inappropriate triggering of perception or memory, without corresponding environmental stimulation. The language production of people with **mania** resembles that seen in receptive aphasia. Emotional reactions after **stroke** differ depending on the location of the damage. Right hemisphere strokes lead to euphoria or unconcern; left hemisphere lesions commonly produce depression, implying that emotions, or the inhibition of emotions, are partly lateralized in the human brain.

The strongest correlations between brain function and psychiatric disorders occur in **schizophrenia** and **obsessive-compulsive disorder**. Prefrontal activity is increased in patients with obsessive compulsive-disorder, who are overly abstract and given to excessive planning. By contrast, PET scans have uncovered decreased functioning of the prefrontal cortex in some schizophrenic patients with negative symptoms like apathy, paucity of speech, flat affect, and difficulty sustaining attention. Enlargement of cerebral ventricles is another well-validated neuroimaging finding in schizophrenia.

Schizophrenic patients with largely negative symptoms also perform poorly on tests of prefrontal cortical function. These include the **Wisconsin Card-Sorting Test** (WCST), the **Porteus Maze Test** (PMT) and **Continuous Performance Testing** (CPT). The WCST requires patients to organize cards of different color, form and number into different groups. It tests abstraction and the ability to shift response sets. The test is markedly abnormal in people with prefrontal damage. The PMT requires advance planning, which those with prefrontal lesions are unable to do. The CPT, in which patients tap their fingers in response to a letter embedded in series of letters, requires sustained attention. It can be done at the bedside and is another useful test of the integrity of the prefrontal cortex.

Items 28-40

Match the neurotransmitters in the items with the subcortical cluster of cell bodies (nuclei) in the answers below that produce the enzymes necessary for the synthesis of these transmitters. Answers may be used once, more than once, or not at all.

(A) Substantia nigra, ventral tegmentum
(B) Raphe (midline and dorsal) of brainstem
(C) Locus ceruleus
(D) Nucleus basalis of Meynert

28. serotonin (5-HT)

29. acetylcholine (ACH)

30. norepinephrine (NE)

31. dopamine (DA)

Choose the **BEST** response.

32. In the normal brain, DA is thought to be involved in

   (A) movement
   (B) sleep
   (C) reward, motivation
   (D) A and C only
   (E) A, B, and C

33. In the normal brain, 5-HT appears to be involved in

   (A) feeding, sleep, temperature
   (B) aggression, motivation
   (C) memory
   (D) A and B only
   (E) A, B, and C

34. The disease process most clearly linked to degeneration of ACH neurons and loss of ACH function in the brain is

   (A) dementia of the Alzheimer's type
   (B) dementia syndrome of depression
   (C) dementia secondary to Parkinson's disease
   (D) deficit state of schizophrenia
   (E) Huntington's disease

35. In parallel with diminished ACH activity, the disorder in Item 34 is characterized by

   (A) decreased norepinephrine (NE) activity
   (B) decreases in central somatostatin and corticotropin (ACTH) activity
   (C) presence of the apolipoprotein E4 gene
   (D) A and C only
   (E) A, B, and C

36. The characteristic pathological changes of the disorder in Item 34 include all the following **EXCEPT**:

   (A) cell loss
   (B) amyloid deposition
   (C) neurofibrillary tangles
   (D) granulovascular degeneration of neurons
   (E) dendritic proliferation

37. DA is centrally involved in the pathophysiology of all of the following conditions **EXCEPT**:

(A) schizophrenia
(B) mania
(C) dementia of the Alzheimer's type
(D) attention-deficit/hyperactivity disorder
(E) cocaine abuse, dependence

38. Parkinson's disease and the extrapyramidal side-effects of DA blocking, antipsychotic drugs, are specifically related to decreased activity in the

(A) nigrostriatal pathway
(B) mesolimbic pathway
(C) mesocortical pathway
(D) tuberoinfundibular tract

39. Galactorrhea, or inappropriate lactation, occurs as a side-effect of DA blocking drugs because

(A) DA is the prolactin inhibitory factor (PIF).
(B) Blocking of dopamine effects in the nigrostriatal pathway increases dopamine activity in the mesocortical pathway.
(C) The tuberoinfundibular pathway is blocked in proportion to blockade of other DA pathways.
(D) A and C only
(E) None of the above

40. Loss or dysregulation of cortical input from the locus ceruleus is implicated in

(A) dementia of the Alzheimer's type
(B) dementia syndrome of depression
(C) dementia secondary to Parkinson's disease
(D) Creutzfeldt-Jakob disease
(E) None of the above

ANSWERS AND TUTORIAL ON ITEMS 28-40

The answers are: **28-B; 29-D; 30-C; 31-A; 32-D; 33-E; 34-A; 35-E; 36-E; 37-C; 38-A; 39-D; 40-B**. The pattern of subcortical clusters of cell bodies (nuclei) that send axons to multiple areas of the neocortex and other subcortical areas is repeated many times in the organization of the central nervous system. Degeneration or other lesions of these focal brain centers provide unitary etiologies for otherwise confusing patterns of neurologic symptoms and behavioral change. Loss of subcortical input causes widely dispersed brain areas to fail, producing behavioral, cognitive, emotional, and vegetative symptoms and signs. The cell bodies and axonal projections of the serotonin (5-HT), norepinephrine (NE), dopamine (DA) and acetylcholine (ACH) subsystems of the brain have been mapped in recent decades. Recognition of these neurochemical subsystems has greatly furthered understanding of a variety of psychiatric illnesses, especially dementias and psychotic disorders.

A variety of peptide neurotransmitters, including substance P, neurotensin, cholecystokinin, somatostatin, vasopressin and oxytocin, co-occur in monoamine transmitter systems. Less is currently known about the normal and pathological functioning of these substances. Eventually, they may prove to equal monoamine transmitters in pathological significance.

Various psychopathological syndromes related to dysfunction of DA, ACH and NE will be covered below, with reference to their activity in the normal brain. Serotonergic neurons in the midline raphe of the brainstem radiate to the cerebral cortex, hippocampus, hypothalamus, thalamus, septum, amygdala and spinal cord. Thus, **serotonin** (5-HT) is a primary regulator of temperature, feeding, sleep, memory, aggression, and motivation. 5-HT also regulates the activity of other transmitter systems, specifically noradrenergic and dopaminergic. Secondary adrenergic effects partly account for the ability of serotonergic drugs to relieve depression and anxiety.

The monoamine transmitter **dopamine** (DA) plays a role in many psychiatric disorders. The cell bodies of DA synthesizing neurons cluster in the substantia nigra, the ventral tegmental area (VTA), and the arcuate nucleus and periventricular area of the hypothalamus. The projections from the substantia nigra to the striatum (nigrostriatal tracts) regulate movement and, to some extent, mood. **Parkinson's disease** is characterized by loss of DA in the substantia nigra; blockade of DA receptors in the striatum accounts for the extrapyramidal (Parkinsonian) side- effects of antipsychotic drugs. Dementia tends to occur late in the course of Parkinson's disease, indicating a role for dopamine in cognition as well.

Dopamine receptor (D_2) blockade in the mesolimbic and mesocortical pathways originating in the VTA contributes to the effect of antipsychotic (DA receptor blocking) drugs. This finding has, in circular fashion, contributed to the recognition that abnormalities in dopaminergic pathways are part of all psychotic illnesses, including **schizophrenia**.

Projections of the mesolimbic pathway to the nucleus accumbens subserve the sensation of reward. **Cocaine** and amphetamine exert their effects in part by increasing DA activity in this region. These drugs closely mimic the effect of spontaneously occurring mania, suggesting a possible role for DA in the pathogenesis of this condition.

The fourth DA pathway, the **tuberoinfundibular tract**, inhibits prolactin release from the anterior pituitary. The effect of DA blocking drugs on this pathway produces the side-effect of **galactorrhea**.

Acetylcholine (ACH)-responsive (cholinergic) neurons, originating in the **nucleus basalis of Meynert**, fan out through the neocortex. They radiate extensively to the hippocampus. Converging lines of research point to loss of ACH input as the primary biochemical lesion of **Alzheimer's disease** and senile dementia of the Alzheimer's type (SDAT). Brain autopsies in SDAT have found degeneration of nucleus basalis neurons, as well as decreases in ACH and choline acetyltransferase (the enzyme that synthesizes acetylcholine). The cholinergic drugs **physostigmine** and **arecoline** improve cognitive function somewhat, while anticholinergic drugs impair it.

The characteristic lesions of SDAT (plaques, amyloid, neurofibrillary tangles, cell loss, granulovascular degeneration) seem to cluster in the cortical and hippocampal projection areas of subcortical ACH-containing neurons. Although these findings point to a central role for ACH in SDAT, other neurotransmitters, specifically norepinephrine and the peptides somatostatin and corticotropin, are also decreased. The presence of the apolipoprotein **E4 gene** has also been found more frequently in patients with Alzheimer's disease than in controls.

The **dementia syndrome of depression**, formerly called "pseudodementia" because of its partial reversibility, connotes problems of concentration and memory during severe depressive episodes, especially in elderly people. Depression appears related to dysregulation of the norepinephrine (noradrenergic) (NE) pathways originating in the locus ceruleus. The dementia syndrome of depression, then, may reflect the loss of noradrenergic input to the cortex.

Items 41-44

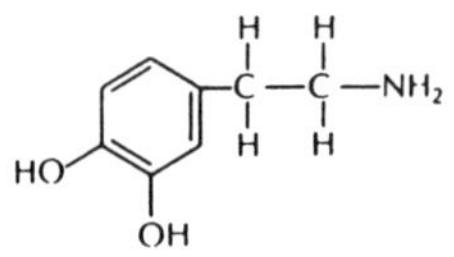

Figure 1.3

41.   The chemical compound shown in Figure 1.3 is

    (A)   epinephrine
    (B)   serotonin
    (C)   dopamine
    (D)   acetylcholine
    (E)   norepinephrine

42.   The main metabolite of this compound is

    (A)   3-methoxy-4-hydroxy-phenylglycol (MHPG)
    (B)   homovanillic acid (HVA)
    (C)   metanephrine
    (D)   5-hydroxyindoleacetic acid (5-HIAA)
    (E)   choline

43.   The main mechanism of clearance of the compound in Figure 1.3 from the synaptic cleft is

    (A)   reuptake into a presynaptic neuron
    (B)   enzymatic degradation in the synaptic cleft
    (C)   enzymatic degradation in the presynaptic neuron
    (D)   diffusion into the extracellular compartment
    (E)   degradation in the postsynaptic neuron

44. The rate limiting enzyme in the biosynthesis of the compound in Figure 1.3 is

    (A)   cathecol-O-methyltransferase
    (B)   tryptophan hydroxylase
    (C)   monoamine A oxidase
    (D)   dopamine-β-hydroxylase
    (E)   tyrosine hydroxylase

ANSWERS AND TUTORIAL ON ITEMS 41-44

The answers are: **41-C; 42-B; 43-A; 44-E**. The compound in **Figure 1.3** is **dopamine**. It is metabolized by monoamine oxidase to form 3,4-dihydroxyphenylglycol (DOPAC) which is subsequently broken down by catechol-O-methyltransferase to its end-product, homovanillic acid. The main mechanism of degradation of dopamine as well as other catecholamines is through reuptake into the presynaptic neuron, where enzymatic breakdown takes place. The rate limiting step in the synthesis of dopamine, epinephrine, and norepinephrine is the conversion of tyrosine to levodopa by the enzyme tyrosine hydroxylase. Aromatic L-amino acid decarboxylase converts levodopa to dopamine. The action of dopamine-β-hydroxylase is responsible for the formation of norepinephrine, which is further converted to epinephrine by the enzyme phenylethanolamine-N-methyl-transferase.

Items 45-48

Choose the **BEST** response.

45. The usual therapeutic dose or potency of typical antipsychotic drugs correlates **BEST** with

    (A)   ability to block D_2 receptors
    (B)   ability to block D_1 receptors
    (C)   ability to block D_3 receptors
    (D)   ratio of D_1 to D_2 receptor blockade

46. Drugs are **BEST** screened for antipsychotic effects by which of the following

    (A)   blockade of apomorphine effects
    (B)   blockade of amphetamine effects
    (C)   induction of catalepsy in rats
    (D)   A and C only
    (E)   A, B, and C

47. The novel antipsychotic clozapine **MOST** differs from earlier dopamine blocking drugs in its

    (A)   increased antagonism of D_1 receptor function
    (B)   high affinity for D_4 receptors
    (C)   ability to antagonize $5\text{-}HT_2$ receptors
    (D)   A and C only
    (E)   A, B, and C

48. The advantages of drugs like clozapine include all the following **EXCEPT**:

    (A)   minimal anticholinergic and antihistaminic effects
    (B)   decreased likelihood of drug induced extrapyramidal side-effects
    (C)   increased efficacy for the negative symptoms of schizophrenia
    (D)   efficacy in patients resistant to older antipsychotic agents
    (E)   decreased likelihood of causing tardive dyskinesia

ANSWERS AND TUTORIAL ON ITEMS 45-48

The answers are: **45-A; 46-E; 47-E; 48-A**. The earliest antipsychotic drug, **chlorpromazine**, was discovered accidentally. Investigation of its effects eventually led to the recognition that drugs that show high affinity for D_2 **dopamine receptors**, which are especially dense in the nigrostriatal pathway, have antipsychotic efficacy. Drugs are screened for their D_2 blocking effects by their ability to antagonize the effects of **apomorphine** and **amphetamine** and their ability to induce **catalepsy** (loss of motor function without loss of consciousness) in rats. The greater the affinity of a drug for the D_2 receptor, the smaller the dose needed to reduce psychotic symptoms and the greater the likelihood of extrapyramidal side-effects or EPSE, e.g., drug-induced parkinsonism, dystonias, and tardive dyskinesia.

Recently, researchers have developed drugs that relieve psychosis by alternate mechanisms. **Clozapine** differs from earlier agents in having little affinity for D_2 receptors and higher affinity for D_1 and D_4 receptors. It also antagonizes the serotonergic $5\text{-}HT_2$ receptor, muscarinic acetylcholine receptors, α_1-**adrenergic** receptors and histaminergic H_1 receptors. This receptor profile produces a novel clinical profile of ability to reduce psychotic symptoms with little likelihood of EPSE. Clozapine is also more effective for negative symptoms like apathy, paucity of speech and mental blankness. Like chlorpromazine, it has marked anticholinergic and some antiadrenergic effects, for example, sedation, hypotension, tachycardia, constipation, weight gain and increased salivation (sialorrhea). An association with lethal **agranulocytosis** in a small number of patients has limited widespread use of clozapine, which is currently given only to patients who have not responded to conventional treatment and who can have their leucocyte counts measured weekly. However, the newer agent **olanzapine** has a similar clinical profile without the risk of agranulocytosis and is likely to be widely used.

Items 49 and 50

Choose the **BEST** response.

49.   Drugs that block the reuptake of norepinephrine and/or serotonin

      (A)   have the potential to induce anxiety
      (B)   may improve depression
      (C)   lead to down regulation of β-adrenergic receptors
      (D)   A and C only
      (E)   A, B, and C

50.   Benzodiazepine drugs given to relieve anxiety and/or induce sleep (sedative hypnotics)

      (A)   augment the activity of γ-amino butyric acid (GABA) via blockade of the coupled benzodiazepine binding site
      (B)   are analeptic in large doses
      (C)   induce tolerance and are associated with withdrawal symptoms, creating significant abuse potential
      (D)   A and C only
      (E)   A, B, and C

ANSWERS AND TUTORIAL ON ITEMS 49 AND 50

The answers are: **49-E; 50-D**. The ability of drugs to relieve depression, anxiety and insomnia has also been correlated with their effects in particular neurotransmitter pathways. Drugs that block the **reuptake of norepinephrine and serotonin** (thereby augmenting their activity upon postsynaptic neurons) are **antidepressants**. In the short-term, they may increase anxiety. Over the course of several weeks, the increase in synaptic transmitter leads to down regulation of postsynaptic β-adrenergic receptors. This effect correlates with the time of onset of antidepressant effects and may be the mechanism by which the drugs improve depressive symptoms.

     Benzodiazepine drugs relieve anxiety and induce and maintain sleep through potentiation of the effects of the inhibitory neurotransmitter γ-amino butyric acid (GABA). The effects of these drugs are immediate. In addition to calming effects, they raise the seizure threshold.

Longer acting benzodiazepines are used as anticonvulsants (the opposite of analeptics). However, over time, people may become tolerant to the therapeutic effects of benzodiazepines, requiring higher and higher doses. Abrupt withdrawal of these drugs leads to rebound anxiety, arousal and insomnia. Both tolerance and the presence of a withdrawal syndrome increase the likelihood that patients will abuse these drugs.

Notes

Notes

CHAPTER II
PERSONALITY DEVELOPMENT,
PSYCHOLOGICAL DEFENSES,
AND SOCIAL ROLE

Items 51-57

Match the names of the scientists with the concepts that they developed. Answers may be used once, more than once, or not at all.

     (A)   Erik Erikson
     (B)   Ivan Pavlov
     (C)   Konrad Lorenz
     (D)   John Bowlby
     (E)   Sigmund Freud
     (F)   Jean Piaget
     (G)   Emil Kraepelin
     (H)   Adolf Meyer
     (I)   Carl Jung
     (J)   Harry Harlow
     (K)   B.F. Skinner

51.   Developed a concept of psychic organization which contained id, ego, and superego.

52.   Studied attachment processes in monkeys including the effects of isolation and separation.

53.   The author of classical conditioning theory.

54.   Ethologist whose studies of imprinting in goslings led to understanding of human bonding behavior.

55.   British psychoanalyst who postulated stages of attachment in human infants.

56.   Studied cognitive organization in children and adults describing sensorimotor, preoperational, concrete operational and formal operational stages.

57.   Described stages of psychosocial development through the life cycle.

ANSWERS AND TUTORIAL ON ITEMS 51-57

The answers are: **51-E; 52-J; 53-B; 54-C; 55-D; 56-F; 57-A**. Behavioral science in medicine concerns those theories which describe or explain human beings at the level of the whole person, in health or normality and when ill. Human subjectivity and behavior have biological, psychological and social determinants, each creating a domain of scientific inquiry. These differing ways of approaching people cannot always be reconciled or reduced into a unitary and universal theory of human functioning. Different theories are still taught as separate, internally consistent paradigms applicable to particular situations or problems. For historical reasons, certain models, especially psychoanalysis, ethology, and behaviorism, have had the greatest impact on physicians' understanding of patients, though none provide an overarching, comprehensive theory that all accept.

The earliest and still most influential modern theory of human functioning, at least in medicine, is psychoanalysis and its derivatives. **Sigmund Freud's** (E) **structural model** of human psychology, one of several created in the early part of this century, organizes mental functions into three parts: **id, ego and superego**. Each component of the mind in Freud's system is responsible for different functions in the psychological life of an individual. The Freudian id is the seat of unconscious impulses and drives, such as love and aggression. The ego exerts executive function in deciding which id impulses can be gratified without untoward effects on the individual's social standing. Freud's superego encompasses parental attitudes, societal norms of behavior, and notions of morality. All these constituents of the mind are largely unconscious and do not correspond to any particular anatomic region of the brain. Freud constructed a conceptual model in order to understand the psychological functioning of individuals. Freud's theories have been particularly influential in leading to the recognition of **defenses**, psychological processes that help people modulate or synthesize competing biological, psychological and social pressures into a coherent self with the ability to behave in organized and adaptive ways. Freud also proposed a model of early human development that progresses through predictable **psychosexual stages**. His concepts of defenses and psychosexual maturation contribute to current models of childhood psychopathology (Chapter IV) and adult personality disorder (Chapter IX).

The study of ethology has become critical in understanding the "nature vs. nurture" controversy in human behavior. Thus Harlow demonstrated an "innate" period after birth which is crucial if **attachment** is to take place. Austrian ethologist **Konrad Lorenz** (C) studied **imprinting** in goslings. He found that shortly after birth, goslings are programmed to follow a moving object, most often the mother. Understanding the "innate" biological mechanisms responsible for bonding, which were first studied in animals, later led to the discovery of endogenous opiates as mediators of **bonding** behavior in humans.

John Bowlby (D), a British psychoanalyst, described the stages of **attachment in infants**. His theory encompasses the description of what attachment is and how it develops. Bowlby also described the anxiety associated with a break in attachment, as in separation of the infant from its mother. Simply stated, **attachment** is an emotional state existing between a child and its caretaker. This emotional state is characterized by the pleasure and soothing that a child experiences with a caretaker. The signs of attachment, such as clinging, seeking out and being pacified by the caretaker, appear as early as 1 month and are present in both humans and nonhuman primates. Disruption of attachment leads to **separation anxiety**, which appears most prominently between 9 and 18 months. Secure attachment in infancy and early childhood is crucial for further development of a healthy person. Severe disruption of early attachments (e.g., by maternal death or depression) may contribute to severe psychopathology in adulthood.

Harry Harlow (J) is known for studies in monkeys on the effects of **social isolation and separation** from a mother figure. In a famous series of experiments, Harlow allowed monkeys who were removed from mothers at birth to seek comfort from either a terry cloth surrogate monkey which provided no food or a wire surrogate monkey which delivered food. Isolated monkeys invariably preferred a terry cloth surrogate, demonstrating an innate need for contact comfort. He also demonstrated that there is a critical period in development, for primates from birth to 6 months, beyond which attachment to a mother figure is not possible. Additionally, Harlow noted that monkeys raised in social isolation without a mother never developed social skills, were unable to mate, and if impregnated, were unable to mother their offspring. Harlow's studies have contributed to the understanding of various psychological and behavioral disorders in infants and children. (Chapter IV)

Russian physiologist **Ivan Pavlov** (B) formulated **classical conditioning theory**. Pavlov studied the salivation response in dogs. Normally, when presented with food, dogs begin to salivate. The food, in this case, is termed an **unconditioned stimulus**, and the salivation is an **unconditioned response**. Having established a pattern of response to the presentation of food, Pavlov coupled a ringing bell with food presentation. Eventually dogs began to associate the sound of the bell with the appearance of food. While bell ringing in itself did not produce salivation, after coupling it with food, dogs began to salivate when hearing the bell in the absence of food. Hence, the bell is a **conditioned stimulus** and salivation, in this case, became a **conditioned response**. **Classical conditioning** applies particularly to responses of the autonomic nervous system, contributing to our understanding of anxiety and anxiety disorders (Chapter IX).

Classical conditioning concerns the animal as a passive object shaped by external forces. **Operant conditioning**, described by **B.F. Skinner** (K), is a more dynamic behavioral model, in which a person or animal acts on the environment, experiences a response, and then responds with a change in subsequent behavior. Operant conditioning partly explains how people learn complex behaviors that go well beyond simple physiological reactions to stimuli. Operant conditioning provides the theoretical framework for behavior therapy, covered in Chapter XI.

Ethology and conditioning theories, while useful, are reductionistic, and do not capture fully the unique aspects of human mental functioning and the human social world. Two perspectives that address these gaps in our understanding are studies of human cognitive development, beginning with the work of Swiss psychologist **Jean Piaget** (F), and **Erik Erikson's** (A) modification of Freud's theory of psychosexual development to include socio-cultural influences.

Piaget closely observed small children to learn how they think. He described how children progress from **sensorimotor** experience of the world to active, patterned modes of reasoning about their experience. He further divided such reasoning into sequential **stages of preoperational, concrete and formal operational thought**. From his careful observations, Piaget developed the **theory of cognitive organization in children and adults**. Piaget further described two ways of thinking about the world that changed as the child developed. Piaget described cognitive organization as **adaptation** to the surrounding world. It consists of two processes, **assimilation** and **accommodation**. In the process of assimilation, new sensory inputs are taken in and simply stored in memory. Accommodation requires that internal thinking change to account for divergent reality.

Erik Erikson (A) has added an important dimension to Freud's psychosexual developmental theory by introducing the **social realm** in which the development of any individual takes place. Erikson believed that we are all social beings whose character is shaped by the culture in which we live. Additionally, Erikson saw development as an ongoing process which does not stop at adolescence. He described life as an orderly succession of psychosocial stages, each characterized by a particular set of conflicts or polarizing forces. People are impelled from one stage to the next by both biological changes (especially in the earliest and latest phases when the rate of biological change is most rapid) and by critical challenges or **crises** created by the competing social pressures of each stage. Failure to resolve the crisis of a particular stage, Erikson stated, affects the individual's ability to confront and resolve the challenges of the next stage, creating lasting patterns of maladaption. Erikson's stages provide a yardstick for relating people's behavior to a standard of normality, helping clinicians differentiate expectable, transient states of distress and dysfunctional behavior from the serious and persistent dysfunctions of psychiatric disorders.

Choose the **BEST** response.

58. Which of the following is the correct order of psychosexual developmental stage postulated by Freud?

    (A)   anal, oral, phallic, latency and genital
    (B)   latency, oral, anal, phallic and genital
    (C)   genital, phallic, oral, anal and latency
    (D)   phallic, anal, oral, latency and genital
    (E)   oral, anal, phallic, latency and genital

59. All of the following are **TRUE** of latency **EXCEPT**:

    (A)   It is the period of rapid hormonal changes and growth spurt in boys.
    (B)   It is a period corresponding to Erikson's crisis of industry vs. inferiority.
    (C)   It is a period of relative quiescence of sexual drives and greater focus on the development of work habits.
    (D)   During this period, the child generally enters the school system, where peer interaction becomes important.
    (E)   During this period, consolidation of gender identity and understanding of sexual roles occurs.

60. Which of the following **BEST** describes Freud's oral stage of development?

    (A)   Corresponds to Piaget's preoperational stage.
    (B)   Spans from birth until approximately 18 months and is marked by use of the mouth as a way of gratifying needs and reducing tension.
    (C)   Is not characterized by aggressive actions of the infant such as biting, chewing, and spitting.
    (D)   . Learning how to talk and express oneself vocally is a major part of this stage.
    (E)   In the first half of this stage, the infant grows to appreciate the mother as a complete and separate being with her own needs and interests.

61. Margaret Mahler's observations of children from birth to age 3 highlighted

    (A)   That a stable mothering figure is important to cognitive as well as emotional development.

    (B)   Conflict in young children over independence vs. the need for adult help.

    (C)   Anxiety, first upon encountering figures who are not the mother (stranger anxiety) and then upon realizing that mother is not present (separation anxiety).

    (D)   A and C only

    (E)   A, B, and C

62. At what age, according to Mahler's observations, might it be **MOST** disruptive to subject an infant to an elective surgical procedure that will require immobilization of the legs

    (A)   4 months

    (B)   8 months

    (C)   16 months

    (D)   36 months

63. Erikson described eight stages of psychosocial behavior. Choose the order in which they occur.

    (A)   trust vs. mistrust, autonomy vs. shame, initiative vs. guilt, industry vs. inferiority, intimacy vs. isolation, generativity vs. stagnation, identity vs. role diffusion, integrity vs. despair.

    (B)   trust vs. mistrust, initiative vs. guilt, autonomy vs. shame, industry vs. inferiority, identity vs. role diffusion, intimacy vs. isolation, generativity vs. stagnation, integrity vs. despair.

    (C)   trust vs. mistrust, autonomy vs. shame, initiative vs. guilt, industry vs. inferiority, identity vs. role diffusion, intimacy vs. isolation, generativity vs. stagnation, integrity vs. despair.

    (D)   trust vs. mistrust, identity vs. role diffusion, autonomy vs. shame, industry vs. inferiority, initiative vs. guilt, intimacy vs. isolation, generativity vs. stagnation, integrity vs. despair.

    (E)   trust vs. mistrust, autonomy vs. shame, initiative vs. guilt, industry vs. inferiority, intimacy vs. isolation, identity vs. role diffusion, generativity vs. stagnation, integrity vs. despair.

64. During which of the following stages does Oedipal conflict take place?

   (A) preoperational
   (B) genital
   (C) initiative vs. guilt
   (D) A and C only
   (E) A, B, and C

65. Which of the following statements **BEST** describes early adulthood?

   (A) Intimacy vs. isolation spans 20-40 years of age.
   (B) The major tasks during this stage are to establish family and career.
   (C) Successful resolution of the crisis of this stage contributes to the individual's productivity and ability to form close, intimate, and exclusive ties with another person.
   (D) Failure to resolve the crisis of this stage results in withdrawal from others and a belief in the malevolence of the world.
   (E) All of the above.

ANSWERS AND TUTORIAL ON ITEMS 58-65

The answers are: **58-E; 59-A; 60-B; 61-E; 62-C; 63-C; 64-D; 65-E**. The task of creating a theoretical model of normal human functioning necessarily involves describing or explaining the steps or transformations that must occur between infancy and adult life. A variety of competing models describe the stages of human development, especially during childhood and adolescence, each from a slightly different point of view. While the theories occasionally contradict or differ from one another, all identify major changes in physical, emotional, and cognitive functioning that occur rapidly between birth and age six or seven, slow down in middle childhood, and accelerate in adolescence, prior to more static adulthood. These **stage theories** have important clinical applications in pediatrics and child psychiatry (see Chapter IV).

Sigmund Freud, who is considered the founder of classic psychoanalysis, described five stages of **psychosexual development: oral, anal, phallic, latency,** and **genital**. He believed that instinctual drives, such as love and aggression, shape the formation of human character. In the process of development, the focus of pleasurable sensation shifts from the mouth (0-2 years) to the anus (2-3 years) and then to the genital area (3-6 years). During the stage of latency, there is a period of sexual quiescence which is disrupted by the onset of puberty (11-13 years). Puberty heralds entry into the adult genital stage.

It is during **latency** that children in Western cultures enter school. The acquisition of **work habits**, the joy of being industrious, and formation of **gender roles** all take place during this time. Peers become extremely important in the process of definition of gender roles. Failure to establish a sense of competence during this time leads to chronic feelings of inferiority and inadequacy.

During the **oral stage** of development spanning the first 18 months of life, the infant learns to experience pleasure through mouth and skin by taking food, calming down with skin contact, sucking on the nipple, etc. This phase corresponds roughly to Piaget's **sensorimotor stage** since the major mode of learning about the world is through the organs of sensation. While the mouth is the major zone of experience for the infant, acquisition of speech as a tool of communication does not take place until age 2. Additionally, while sucking and taking in predominate during the early oral phase, biting as an expression of aggression appears near the end of the stage.

Freud developed his theory about the stages of childhood from watching his own family and from reconstructing patients' histories during the course of psychoanalysis. Although influenced by theory, **Margaret Mahler** described human psychological development based more upon the direct observation of children and caretakers between birth and age 36 months. This period corresponds to the oral and anal psychosexual stages, the psychosocial stages of trust vs. mistrust and autonomy vs. shame and doubt, and the sensorimotor and early preoperational phases of cognitive development. Mahler described how infants progress from a state of symbiotic dependence on a mother to a sense of themselves as separate beings **(separation-individuation)**. She identified several subphases in this process, including cognitive maturation around 8 months of age that allows the infant to recognize the difference between familiar and unfamiliar faces, which engenders a blend of fear and curiosity she termed **stranger anxiety.** Slightly later, around 10 to 16 months, the development of walking leads to repeated experiences of separation from the primary caretaker, to which the child responds with **separation anxiety.** Although locomotion leads to separation, it also produces frequent reunions, contributing to the subphase of **rapprochement** (16-24 months), in which children express the desire to explore while responding to limits, soothing and protection from their caretakers. Finally, Mahler noted that by age 3 children become much more tolerant of separation from caretakers, because they can accept reassurance in language and have the cognitive capacity to recognize that other people do not vanish during times of separation and will return **(object constancy)**.

Mahler's observations suggest that immobilizing the legs of a child younger than a year will be less disruptive than restricting mobility between 12 and 24 months, when so much normal cognitive and emotional development is tied to the development of walking and the ability to be physically separate from caretaking adults for increasing periods of time. By age 36 months, although restriction of mobility might cause considerable distress, a child can better handle frustration through language and can draw upon other skills that will allow development to proceed along its normal path.

Erikson described the formation of individual character against the background of social tasks that the developing person must meet. These stages consist of **crises** that must be resolved for successful maturation. Lack of resolution of a particular crisis, while it does not arrest the development of an individual, "scars" the person and remains as a pattern of maladjustment. The stages he described are: basic trust vs. basic mistrust (0-1 yo), autonomy vs. shame and doubt (1-3 yo), initiative vs. guilt (3-5 yo), industry vs. inferiority (6-11 yo), identity vs. role diffusion (11 yo-end of adolescence), intimacy vs. isolation (21-40 yo), generativity vs. stagnation (40-65 yo) and integrity vs. despair (>65 yo).

Oedipal conflict, simply defined by a child falling in love with the parent of the opposite sex and fearing retaliation for such feelings from the parent of the same sex, takes place during Freud's **phallic stage** of psychosexual development, which chronologically corresponds to Piaget's **preoperational stage** (ages 2-7) and Erikson's **initiative vs. guilt**. In the stage of initiative, the child is actively curious about his/her genitals and those of others. Parental and societal attitudes discouraging such explorations can lead to feelings of guilt. During the genital stage, adult sexuality is established and Oedipal conflict is, in theory, resolved.

Erikson's stage of **intimacy vs. isolation** spans from early to middle adulthood (21-40 yo). During this time, most adults establish careers and family, which leads to the sense of productivity. Relationships with people deepen and reinforce the perception of others as helpful and well-meaning. Failure to resolve the crisis of this stage leads to withdrawal from social interactions and the impression of the world as a cruel and lonely place.

Items 66-69

Tommy is a 4-year-old boy who is generally happy and well-adjusted. His parents consult a pediatrician because they recently became concerned with the boy's behavior. Tommy is found to touch his genitals incessantly. He is very curious when his 18-month-old baby sister gets a diaper change. Yesterday he asked his mother what happened to his sister's penis and confided to his mother that when Daddy leaves on his business trip, Tommy will marry his mother.

66.   Your **BEST** response to the parents' questions should be

(A)   Tommy's increased sexual behavior strongly suggests sexual molestation. Parents should question the babysitter about her sexual contact with Tommy.

(B)   Tommy feels a lack of parental interest because of the presence of his little sister and engages in provocative behavior to keep his parents' attention on himself.

(C)   Tommy is developing prematurely and beginning to exhibit sexuality commonly found in the genital stage of development.

(D)   Tommy's behavior is quite normal and consistent with Erikson's stage of initiative vs. guilt. He is active, happy and curious, especially in sexual matters.

(E)   His desire to marry his mother and avoid imagined punishment by his father demonstrates that his parents were especially strict in his earlier development.

67.   Your **BEST** recommendation would be

(A)   Ignore the behavior, it will likely disappear.
(B)   Encourage Tommy's curiosity, answer questions about sexual anatomy simply and matter-of-factly, and avoid shaming.
(C)   Make an appointment for evaluation by a child psychiatrist to prevent development of further problems.
(D)   Tell Tommy to stop touching himself because "others will laugh at him". Do not change his little sister in his presence.
(E)   Tell Tommy that he and his mother will get married when he grows up, but for now he has to wait.

68.   To what stage of development does Tommy's behavior correspond?

(A)   phallic
(B)   autonomy vs. shame and doubt
(C)   preoperational
(D)   A and C
(E)   A, B, and C

69.   Various tasks at this stage of Tommy's development include

(A)   Learning by copying the world of adults, i.e., pretending to go to work.
(B)   Identification with the same sex parent upon resolution of Oedipal conflict, i.e., "shaving" like the father.
(C)   Learning the positive value of curiosity even if it is initially intrusive to others.
(D)   A and C only
(E)   A, B, and C

ANSWERS AND TUTORIAL ON ITEMS 66-69

The answers are: **66-D; 67-B; 68-D; 69-E**. Tommy's behavior is typical of a child between ages 3 and 5. He is curious, especially in sexual self-exploration. His curiosity about his sister's genitals is consistent with trying to differentiate between boys and girls. While **sexually molested children** may exhibit hypersexual behavior, they also frequently show disturbance of mood, delay in reaching developmental milestones, and general mistrust of adults. While **sibling rivalry** is common at this stage and may present itself by children fighting to gain parental attention even to the point of the older harming the younger sibling, it is unusual to present itself with increased sexual curiosity. There is no evidence that Tommy's behavior is premature. The **adult genital stage** is marked by **mutual** sexual interest and the search for a reasonable sexual partner which obviously does not include one's parents. Tommy's desire to marry his mother and his fear of his father is typical of the Oedipal complex and is normal between the ages of 3 and 7.

Ignoring Tommy's behavior gives him the message that his parents are uncomfortable with his sexuality and are not able to discuss it rationally. During this time, avoiding **shaming** is of paramount importance, since the child's experience of his body as good and competent plays a critical role in the later development of self-esteem and pride in accomplishment. Since Tommy's behavior is normal and age appropriate, no consultation with a child psychiatrist is needed. It is harmful for a child to be supported in his fantasy of marrying a parent. A gentle statement of "When you grow up you'll marry somebody like your mother" is more reasonable.

Tommy's behavior is clearly indicative of the **phallic stage** based on his curiosity about his own and his sister's genitals and preoccupation with Oedipal matters. This corresponds chronologically to **Piaget's preoperational stage**. The preoperational stage of **cognitive development** is characterized by lack of causal and logical thinking and inability to classify objects. Children tend to be self-centered, think in magical terms, and begin to use language symbolically. Autonomy vs. shame precedes Tommy's current stage of development. Social tasks that Tommy must master during the initiative vs. guilt stage include identification with the same sex parent, learning about the world by copying the actions of adults, and learning the positive value of curiosity.

Items 70-72

Liz is a 15-year-old female. She does reasonably well in school and has a few good friends. Her parents are concerned that Liz is headed for trouble ever since they discovered that she had been drinking at a girlfriend's party.

70. Drinking and using drugs at this stage

    (A)   Is a normal part of adolescent experimentation.

    (B)   Strongly predicts adult abuse of drugs and alcohol.

    (C)   Should be strictly prohibited as it is illegal.

    (D)   Should be brought to the attention of the school, Liz's pediatrician and legal authorities.

    (E)   Should be discussed with Liz by pointing out that it is illegal and potentially harmful to her health. Parents should investigate with her what motivates her to drink with friends at the party.

71. Her parents have noted that Liz becomes moody, hides in her room listening to hard rock, worships the latest rock singer, and acts in a condescending manner toward her parents, saying that they are boring. Your understanding of Liz's behavior is

    (A)   Liz is in the midst of a depressive episode. Tricyclic antidepressants are recommended.

    (B)   In the process of identity formation, Liz's identity has changed completely to the opposite of her parents.

    (C)   Mood swings, isolation and hero worship are common in adolescence.

    (D)   A and C only

    (E)   A, B, and C

72. According to Piaget's theory of cognitive development, all of the following are **TRUE** about Liz **EXCEPT**:

    (A)   Liz is currently entering the stage of formal operational thinking.

    (B)   Liz is to be expected to think abstractly, and to be able to use both deductive and inductive reasoning.

    (C)   Moral and ethical considerations are becoming more flexible, governed by relativism and not strict application of rules.

    (D)   This stage is also characterized by phenomenalistic causality and animistic thinking.

    (E)   Language is complex and follows laws of grammar. Sentence structure is logical.

ANSWERS AND TUTORIAL ON ITEMS 70-72

The answers are: **70-E; 71-C; 72-D**. While drinking alcohol and experimentation with drugs are a part of life for many adolescents, completely ignoring it is not prudent. The best approach is for parents to engage in meaningful discussion with the teen, treating him/her like an adult. Discussion of the risks of such behavior invites an adolescent to participate in decision-making concerning his/her life.

During adolescence, mood swings, anxiety states, and periods of circumscribed irrationality are common and do not constitute psychopathology. It is during these periods that a teenager attempts to define him/herself. Hero worship, stronger peer identification, and rebellion against parental values all contribute to the formation of unique individual personality.

Interestingly, upon resolution of the adolescent crisis, most teenagers retain a large portion of their parents' identity and values.

The stage of **formal operational thinking** is characterized by burgeoning ability to abstract, to manipulate complicated problems, to use deductive and inductive reasoning, and to use language skillfully and extensively. Morality is guided by personal ethical convictions and not by strict application of societal rules. **Phenomenalistic causality**, which is defined by the belief that events occurring simultaneously or in close succession cause each other, is characteristic of the **preoperational stage**. Likewise **animistic** thinking, defined as the attribution of psychological states and feelings to inanimate objects, occurs during the preoperational stage.

Items 73-77

Match the developmental stages in the answers to the statements that **BEST** describe them in the items below. Answers may be used once, more than once, or not at all.

(A)   Oral stage
(B)   Preoperational stage
(C)   Sensorimotor stage
(D)   Anal stage
(E)   Phallic stage
(F)   Concrete operational stage
(G)   Intimacy vs. isolation

73.   John is 4 years old. He believes that thinking about snow will make it come and that his teddy bear feels pain when dropped.

74.   Anne is 24 years old. She has received her graduate degree and settled in the career of mechanical engineer. She is still looking for "that special man".

75.   Stubbornness and fastidiousness may become lifelong traits during this period.

76.   The child receives particular pleasure from sucking, chewing and biting.

77.   Jeff, who is 3 1/2 years old, loves to take his clothes off, especially when company arrives, and perform various dances for adults.

ANSWERS AND TUTORIAL ON ITEMS 73-77

The answers are: **73-B; 74-G; 75-D; 76-A; 77-E**. John demonstrates thinking consistent with the **preoperational stage** (B). His belief in causing a snowfall demonstrates both **egocentric and magical thinking**, so prominent at this age. **Animistic thought** is evident in John's belief that his teddy bear has feelings. Although chronologically John falls into the phallic stage (E), typical "phallic" behavior is not described.

Anne is negotiating Erikson's **intimacy vs. isolation crisis** (G). During this time, which spans from early to middle adulthood, people settle on a career and look to establish a family.

The **anal stage** (D) is marked by increased control over muscle sphincters and pleasure associated with either withholding or letting go. The child, for the first time, realizes that he/she can make parents happy by being clean and producing a bowel movement or frustrated by withholding or being messy. Difficulties in resolving these opposing attitudes, especially where toilet training is particularly strict, may result in a lifelong pattern of stubbornness, fastidiousness or messiness.

Pleasure that is located in the oral zone and is expressed through licking, sucking, chewing or biting is typical of the **oral stage** (A). Additionally, other experiences represented by passive taking in, such as being touched, caressed, seeing and hearing are important means of reducing tension at this stage.

Jeff demonstrates behavior of a child in the **phallic stage** (E). He has discovered his genitals and his body. Finding such a discovery pleasing, he is happy to share it with others. Showing off other accomplishments, such as improved complicated motor control, is quite common for children in this stage.

Items 78-82

Choose the **BEST** response.

78.   All of the following are **TRUE** regarding defense mechanisms **EXCEPT**:

(A)   Defenses originate in the ego and are largely unconscious.
(B)   Only disturbed individuals exhibit ego defense mechanisms.
(C)   Defenses may be narcissistic, immature, neurotic or mature.
(D)   The purpose of defense mechanisms is to protect individuals from the untoward effects of release of instinctual drives.
(E)   Anna Freud was the first to thoroughly study and classify defense mechanisms.

79. All of the following are narcissistic or primitive defense mechanisms **EXCEPT**:

(A) denial
(B) projection
(C) altruism
(D) splitting
(E) idealization

80. A trauma surgeon spent the last twelve hours in surgery assisting the victims of a massive car collision. There were many casualties, and a number of patients died on the operating table. When asked about his day by his wife upon arrival at home, the surgeon proceeds to recount in meticulous detail the events of the preceding twelve hours without any evidence of emotion. The defense mechanism displayed by the surgeon is

(A) projective identification
(B) reaction formation
(C) professionalism
(D) isolation of affect
(E) psychotic denial

81. When confronted by his wife about his seeming lack of feeling while describing such a tragic catastrophe, the surgeon becomes irate, screaming at his wife for annoying him and getting on his nerves after a long day of work. This is an example of

(A) denial
(B) reaction formation
(C) displacement
(D) splitting
(E) rationalization

82. When asked by his colleague the next day about his fight at home, the surgeon proceeds to explain his angry outburst as a rational response to an annoying wife; after all she should know better than to bother him after work. The defense mechanism employed in this case is

(A) rationalization
(B) reaction formation
(C) projective identification
(D) repression
(E) regression

ANSWERS AND TUTORIAL ON ITEMS 78-82

The answers are: **78-B; 79-C; 80-D; 81-C, 82-A**. While the first to describe **defense mechanisms** was **Sigmund Freud**, he concentrated his attention largely on **repression**. His daughter, **Anna Freud**, studied the defense mechanisms of the ego in great detail. **George Vaillant** further classified and investigated defense mechanisms in both healthy and ill individuals. Defense mechanisms are functions of the **ego** and are **largely unconscious**. Their purpose is to protect the individual from the awareness of painful feelings or disagreeable thoughts. Mature defenses characterize the functioning of normal individuals. Immature, narcissistic, and neurotic defenses are largely responsible for the presenting symptomatology of many psychiatric syndromes, especially personality disorders. The following are considered narcissistic, or primitive defense mechanisms: **denial, projection, projective identification, primitive idealization**, and **splitting**. Immature defenses include **acting out, somatization, regression**, and **passive-aggression**. Neurotic defenses include **displacement, intellectualization, isolation of affect, repression, reaction formation, rationalization**, and **dissociation**. Finally, mature defenses are: **altruism, humor, sublimation, anticipation**, and **suppression**.

The surgeon, who is able to describe the gruesome details of human suffering without a shred of emotion, is a prime example of defense mechanisms at work. By unconsciously being able to employ the defense of **isolation of affect**, he protects himself from experiencing the excruciating pain involved in witnessing a human catastrophe. In the defense of isolation of affect, the feeling accompanying a thought or experience is split off and repressed. What remains in a person's awareness is only the thought or experience. This type of defense is common among medical personnel and scientists as well as in patients with obsessive-compulsive personality disorder.

However, upon returning home, when stressed further by his wife's well-intentioned inquiry, the pain of recalling the event overwhelms him, and, being unable to isolate affect anymore, he displaces his feelings of anger and outrage onto his wife, thus employing the defense of **displacement**. Displacement frequently operates in "kicking the dog" behaviors. The person, object or situation onto which the original feeling is displaced usually resembles, in some way, the initial situation, but is less threatening in nature.

When further stressed by a colleague's curiosity, our surgeon resorts to **rationalization** to avoid the pain of realizing that he has offended his wife for no good reason. In rationalization, seemingly plausible explanations are used to explain attitudes, feelings or beliefs that are otherwise unacceptable.

Items 83-89

Match the listed defense mechanisms in the answers with the **BEST** description of the behavior, exemplifying the appropriate defenses, in the items below. Answers may be used once, more than once, or not at all.

(A) Splitting
(B) Projection
(C) Repression
(D) Suppression
(E) Reaction formation
(F) Denial
(G) Intellectualization
(H) Sublimation
(I) Altruism
(J) Regression

83. Tony is an artist. He has noticed that most of the time his artistic inspiration comes to him in the moments of despair. He is drawn to his paints and, having finished the piece, feels relieved of sadness.

84. Having overspent money doing holiday shopping, Susan temporarily decides to "forget" a bill, the payment of which is not crucial. Even though Susan does not pay the bill on time, she, nevertheless, periodically recalls the need to pay it eventually.

85. During the course of a protracted illness, Bill, who is otherwise an efficient and competent executive of a large corporation, becomes childlike, refuses to bathe and feed himself, and demands that his wife take over his basic functions, even though he is capable of performing these tasks himself.

86. The famous line from Shakespeare's *Hamlet*, "The lady doth protest too much, methinks", exemplifies this defense mechanism.

87. Dorothy has been experiencing many difficulties in her current relationship with Jack, her boyfriend. She feels extreme attraction for him, and when he satisfies her needs, she feels he is a "knight in shining armor". However, if he is not immediately and readily available, Dorothy becomes irate, despondent and believes Jack to be "the Devil personified".

88. Having suffered much deprivation while growing up, Anne decided to become a social worker so she would be able to assist others in a similar plight.

89. John insists in an angry and combative manner that his coworkers are furious with him and are planning to sabotage his work. His supervisor, looking into this matter, finds no evidence of such behavior and refers John for a psychological evaluation.

ANSWERS AND TUTORIAL ON ITEMS 83-89

The answers are: **83-H; 84-D; 85-J; 86-E; 87-A; 88-I; 89-B**. **Sublimation** (H) is a mature defense mechanism in which painful feelings or experiences are transformed into productive or creative outcomes. This process of transformation brings relief from pain.

Suppression (D) is the only defense mechanism which may be conscious. It allows us to temporarily postpone making a decision, which would potentially involve some psychological distress, such as the realization of having low funds and feeling financially irresponsible. Unlike **repression**, which is entirely unconscious forgetting, suppression does not prevent an individual from carrying out necessary actions at a more opportune time.

Regression (J) is a fairly common phenomenon when dealing with physical illness. As the name implies, it involves the return to earlier stages of development when under stress. Regression protects the individual from the discomfort of accepting adult responsibility and permits the establishment of the **sick role**.

Reaction formation (E) is a neurotic defense mechanism in which an unacceptable impulse is reversed into its opposite. An example, in addition to Gertrude's famous line, would include a lascivious person advocating celibacy as the only moral way of life. A person's apparent ardor in the manifest expression of a belief frequently betrays reaction formation in action.

Splitting (A) is among the most primitive defense mechanisms. It involves an inability to integrate the positive and negative aspects of an individual or a situation into one cohesive whole. Because it operates at a very early developmental stage, splitting prevents the "contamination" of the good by the bad in the developing child. When it persists into adulthood, it manifests itself in extreme views, often about the same individual. It is characteristically present in borderline personality disorder.

In **altruism** (I), one's own individual pain is used to benefit others. It is among the mature defense mechanisms. **Projection** (B) is among the primitive defense mechanisms. It is most active in psychosis and is manifested in delusions and ideas of reference. The person using projection takes painful or unacceptable impulses and attributes them to individuals and circumstances outside of the self. The impulses most often thus attributed are of aggressive or sexual nature.

Items 90-95

Choose the **BEST** response.

90. The structural theory of the mind classifies all of the following as ego functions **EXCEPT**:

    (A) modulation of reactivity to internal and external world (sensory thresholds)
    (B) intelligence, learning and language
    (C) judgment (capacity to predict outcomes and appreciate the consequences of one's actions)
    (D) innate sexual and aggressive impulses
    (E) synthesis of disparate elements (memory, bodily state, perception and belief) into unified, stable representations of self, others, and the material world

91. Psychological defenses and other ego functions are especially relevant to medicine because

    (A) They help explain why the same event may be stressful or pathogenic for one individual and benign for another.
    (B) They provide a means of understanding resilience in the face of adverse experience, explaining how people can remain well despite serious stress.
    (C) They are elements of personality which may be either adaptive or disordered and a focus of clinical intervention.
    (D) A and C only
    (E) A, B, and C

92. Which of the following statements **BEST** describes the relationship between stress and illness?

    (A) The cumulative number of life change units, determined by the weighted scores given on the Holmes Rahe Social Readjustment Scale, predicts whether a person will develop a serious illness in the following year.
    (B) Any amount or pattern of stress predisposes individuals to illness.
    (C) Maturity of defenses, prior experience, habitual optimism or pessimism, and preparedness all affect how stressful a given life event seems to a given person. The meaning the person gives to an event affects its potential to precipitate or exacerbate illness.
    (D) A and C only
    (E) A, B and C

93. The life events requiring the highest levels of readjustment are in **DESCENDING** order

    (A) death of a parent, divorce, death of a child, death of a spouse, marriage, incarceration, serious illness or injury, being fired

    (B) death of a child, death of a spouse, new job, marriage, death of a parent, being fired, incarceration

    (C) death of a spouse, divorce, marital separation, incarceration, death of a close family member, serious illness or injury, marriage, being fired

    (D) divorce, incarceration, being fired, death of a spouse, death of a parent, death of a child, marriage, serious illness

    (E) serious illness, death of a spouse, divorce, incarceration, being fired, marital separation, death of a parent or child

94. Animal models of stress relevant to medical and psychiatric illness include all the following **EXCEPT**:

    (A) learned helplessness
    (B) constant artificial light
    (C) separation of infants from mothers
    (D) chronic crowding, unpredictable feeding and interrupted sleep
    (E) social isolation

95. Stressful experiences may precipitate or contribute to physical illness by

    (A) compromising immune function
    (B) increasing unhealthy behaviors, e.g., smoking, drinking, noncompliance with treatment
    (C) affecting the functioning of the autonomic nervous system
    (D) A and C only
    (E) A, B, and C

ANSWERS AND TUTORIAL ON ITEMS 90-95

The answers are: **90-D; 91-D; 92-D; 93-C; 94-B; 95-E**. The concept of **ego functions** represents a second generation of psychoanalytic theory, beginning with the work of **Anna Freud** and others including **Heinz Hartmann** and **Leo Bellak**. These analysts devoted attention to observable aspects of the whole person, including intelligence, perception, regulation of bodily states (impulses and emotions), judgment, and language. All of these are synthetic functions. The ego combines disparate elements of psychological functioning into relatively stable representations of self and others. For example, drawing upon a range of memories of interpersonal interactions, current and remembered mood, usual defensive repertoire, culturally instilled beliefs, and capacity for problem solving, a person may feel fundamentally worthy and capable. Such a stable self-concept will not dissolve in the face of a recent failure or rejection, though it may require modification over time. In psychoanalytic theory, innate sexual and aggressive impulses or instincts are ascribed to the id, which the ego regulates.

The understanding of **psychological defenses** and other ego functions accounts for much of the variability in human reactions to stress. Early research on stress involved developing a list of common life events and ranking them by the degree to which they require persons to make major changes in thinking or behavior. The standard scale of life events, the Holmes Rahe Social Readjustment Rating Scale, ranks death of a spouse, divorce, marital separation, incarceration, death of a close family member, major injury or illness, getting married, and being fired as the eight most challenging or stressful life events. This ranking underlies the protective or socially supportive effects of close relationships, and the damage caused by their disruption. The number of recent events statistically weighted in this ranking correlates modestly with the development of subsequent physical illness.

The power of events to **predict illness** increases when researchers measure the degree to which the person perceives events as favorable or unfavorable, stressful or not stressful. Stressful events are typically unpredictable or unexpected, have uncontrollable effects, and induce negative emotional reactions. People whose psychological defenses include intellectualization, anticipation, humor, and suppression are able to foresee difficulties, exert some control over their circumstances and maintain a positive (hopeful, cheerful, trusting) psychological/emotional state. These qualities contribute to resilience, the obverse of vulnerability. The concepts of vulnerability and resilience shape professional understanding of the range of people's reactions to experience, including the experience of illness or disease.

Not all **stress** is destructive. Lack of stimulation or challenge can be as debilitating as overwhelming demand. Moderate levels of stress can help people develop a wider and more effective range of coping behaviors, stimulate the maturation of psychological defenses, enhance self-esteem, and develop the capacity to work and form good relationships.

Although resilience and vulnerability may vary during different periods of people's lives or in different contexts, people are typically quite consistent over time, either in their ability to adapt successfully or in proneness to dysphoric emotions, unstable or skewed relationships, inability to accomplish life goals, and maladaptive behaviors. An individual's enduring patterns of mood, defenses, behaviors and modes of relating to others are deemed **personality**. When people show difficulty in these domains over long periods of time in many different contexts, they may be considered to have personality disorders. **Personality disorders** are, in turn, a potential focus of psychiatric intervention, traditionally by psychotherapy but now also by drugs that may modify underlying emotional reactions (see Chapter IX).

Much of the research on stress and medical or psychiatric illness has been done on animals. Various paradigms mimic situations analogous to conditions that humans commonly find stressful. The **learned helplessness model** involves exposing dogs to repeated, inescapable shock. Later, when the means to avoid the shock are provided, the dogs do not learn to escape. Researchers have also studied the nature and duration of the reactions of infant monkeys to various degrees of separation from their mothers. Other studies involve rearing monkeys in isolation and then re-exposing them to others. Rat experiments that involve crowding, sleep disruption, and the unpredictable availability of food provide yet another experimental model of stress. Each of these models evokes responses that correspond to various pathological or maladaptive behaviors in humans, including dysregulations of arousal, inappropriate social behavior, apathy, self-mutilation, self-stimulation, aggression and inability to parent. Continuous exposure to light has been used to study circadian rhythms but is not considered a model of stress.

These animal studies have produced information on the adverse physical effects of different kinds of stress. Various measures of immune function, including lymphocyte counts, T cell activation, and cortisol levels, are affected by stress. These, in turn, may account for some of the relationship between stress and the onset or progression of infections, cancer, or autoimmune diseases.

Stress can lead to chronically increased or dysregulated autonomic arousal, manifested in hypertension, sleep disorders, irritable bowel symptoms, coronary artery disease, and cardiac arrhythmias, including sudden death. Stress typically causes hyperacidity in the stomach and may lead to the development of gastritis and ulcers. In humans, the physical effects of stress may also be exacerbated by increased drinking or smoking.

The potentially therapeutic or meliorative effects of various interventions have also been demonstrated in these animal models. For example, certain monkeys have the capacity to teach peers raised as isolates to play and interact normally. Antidepressants help reverse learned helplessness and can reduce separation distress in animal studies.

Items 96-99

Choose the **BEST** response.

96.   Social role theory

    (A)   Posits patterns of expected attitudes and behaviors (roles) that exist outside of individuals, but are implicit in the way relations between people are organized in a given society.

    (B)   Declares that subjective experiences--self-esteem, anger, sadness, anxiety--often derive, not from past personal experience, but from fit or lack of fit in existing social roles.

    (C)   States that roles are maintained by reciprocal interactions between people and that deviance from a given role will elicit a reaction from others (correction, disapproval, rejection, punishment) meant to restore it.

    (D)   All of the above

    (E)   None of the above

97. As described by Talcott Parsons, the sick role includes all the following parameters **EXCEPT**:

    (A)   The patient is not responsible for becoming ill.
    (B)   The patient temporarily gives up his/her usual responsibilities.
    (C)   The patient must be thoroughly educated about his/her illness.
    (D)   The patient should want to get better.
    (E)   The patient seeks out and complies with treatment.

98. Other true statements about the sick role as defined by Parsons include

    (A)   The sick role receives more support and acceptance when confirmed by a physician than when assumed unilaterally.
    (B)   Society expects people to value the sick role and to adopt it eagerly when appropriate.
    (C)   The sick role evolves over time, through the stages of symptom recognition, assumption of the sick role, contact with medical care, dependent relationship with caretakers, and rehabilitation/recovery.
    (D)   A and C only
    (E)   A, B, and C

99. The psychiatric disorders related to aberrant sick role behavior include all of the following **EXCEPT**:

    (A)   somatization disorder
    (B)   malingering
    (C)   pseudoparkinsonism
    (D)   factitious disorder
    (E)   conversion disorder

Items 100-104

Certain personality traits cause patients to violate the expectations of the sick role and elicit corrective or punitive responses from caretakers, especially in medical settings. Match the personality trait below with the statement about sick role behavior that **BEST** matches it. Answers may be used once, more than once, or not at all.

    (A)   Dependent strivings
    (B)   Antisociality
    (C)   Narcissism
    (D)   Borderline traits
    (E)   Compulsiveness
    (F)   Schizotypy
    (G)   Suspiciousness/mistrust (nonpsychotic paranoia)
    (H)   Passivity
    (I)   Histrionic personality style

100.   Patients exaggerate their complaints but present them so vaguely, physicians doubt they are real.

101.   Patients are reluctant to seek medical care and may have trouble forming an appropriately dependent relationship with a physician or complying with recommendations.

102.   Patients are reluctant to resume normal responsibilities and detach from the role of recipient of care.

103.   Patients have difficulty acknowledging signs of illness in themselves.

104.   Hospital staff often find themselves disagreeing with one another over the legitimacy of the patient's distress; patients may alternate between angry rejection of proffered help and undue passivity or neediness.

ANSWERS AND TUTORIAL ON ITEMS 96-104

The answers are: **96-D; 97-C; 98-D; 99-C; 100-H; 101-G (C, F might also apply); 102-A; 103-C; 104-D**. The **sick role** as defined by **Talcott Parsons** provides a useful way of understanding many of the problems that arise between physicians and patients. Rather than ascribe difficulties to faults or deficits in either person, social role theory, which includes all three statements in Item 96, would question how each individual might be deviating from the expectations of his/her role, and how the other party is attempting to re-establish role appropriate behavior.

The four defining qualities, two rights and two responsibilities, of the sick role are given in Item 97. Although it is desirable to educate patients about their conditions, this is not a necessary aspect of the sick role. Patients need only recognize they are in some way ill. The responsibility for understanding the illness belongs to the doctor role, though the doctor can (and should) share this understanding with the patient.

The sick role is necessary and useful in society, but **undesirable** or deviant. Patients are not fulfilling their normal obligations. They are expected to want to get well and relinquish the sick role as soon as possible. Indeed, the sick role is time-limited. Patients who remain in it too long move into the more devalued **disabled role**. People who are too eager to assume the sick role may be looked down upon as manipulative, malingering, or inadequate. Paradoxically, the sick role is given most readily to patients who are least eager to remain in it for any length of time.

Pseudoparkinsonism is a term describing the thoroughly real extrapyramidal side-effects of dopamine blocking drugs. Aberrant sick role behavior is a part of the other disorders on this list. Factitious disorder describes patients who make themselves ill in order to receive medical care, which gratifies deeply felt, though often disavowed, needs for acceptance, specialness, and legitimacy. People with somatization disorder express ambivalence and emotional distress though various bodily symptoms rather than language. In conversion disorder, patients express a more focal problem, often a response to a traumatic experience, through a single symptom or pattern of symptoms. Neither somatization nor conversion, by definition, can be confirmed as manifestations of illness by physicians, who then refuse to validate the patients in the sick role. Malingering describes patients who assume or remain too long in the sick role to avoid responsibilities.

Any personality trait that people may exhibit is likely to influence their behavior in a given social role. **Histrionic personality style** (I) implies that the person is flamboyant, dramatic, and often seductive or impulsive. Patients with this quality may describe their medical symptoms in dramatic terms, without being able to substantiate them on cross-questioning.

Paranoid patients (G) mistrust physicians. They tend to scrutinize every bit of advice or information they are given, and will often be noncompliant out of fear of unforeseen, negative consequences. **Schizotypal patients** (F) often have idiosyncratic perceptions and odd reasoning that also can impair their ability to understand and follow medical advice. Conversely, patients with deeply felt desires to be cared for by others will readily adopt the sick role when ill. The experience of receiving care may be so gratifying, however, that they have trouble appropriately relinquishing the sick role when they are better.

Narcissistic patients (C) are, by definition, convinced of their own specialness and superior capabilities. Narcissistic people have trouble allowing themselves to be dependent on others out of fear of appearing weak. Signs of illness threaten their sense of being above the normal constraints of life. If they do acknowledge illness, however, they often become very demanding. They may insist that their illness is rare, severe, and special, or become angry if treatment does not lead to perfect restoration of function.

Patients with **borderline personality traits** (D) often manage distress by "splitting"-- oscillating between one feeling and its opposite, without being aware of the incompatibility. They may express anger and resentment to one person and act helpless and deeply appreciative with another. This inconsistency can divide treatment groups into those who respond to the borderline patient's angry, manipulative behavior and those who are privy to the person's underlying distress.

CHAPTER III
EVALUATION, DIAGNOSIS,
AND RISK ASSESSMENT

Items 105 and 106

Choose the **BEST** response.

105. The prevailing diagnostic paradigm in psychiatry, embodied in the Diagnostic and Statistical Manual-IV (DSM-IV), is

   (A)   phenomenological
   (B)   limited to valid disease categories
   (C)   a systematic reconciliation of medical psychiatry and psychoanalysis
   (D)   A and C only
   (E)   A, B, and C

106. The DSM-IV improves on other diagnostic schemes in its

   (A)   construct validity
   (B)   ability to generate meaningful prognoses for all patients
   (C)   reliability and standardization of terms
   (D)   A and C only
   (E)   A, B, and C

ANSWERS AND TUTORIAL ON ITEMS 105 AND 106

The answers are: **105-A; 106-C**. The **Diagnostic and Statistical Manual** (DSM) provides a standardized, phenomenological scheme for classifying disorders with prominent mental or behavioral symptoms. This approach dates back to the work of the German psychiatrist **Emil Kraepelin** (1856-1926), who carefully observed a large number of institutionalized patients over many years and classified them according to the primary symptoms and characteristic courses of their conditions. Such a descriptive scheme does not require that the cause(s) of a particular disorder be known for it to be a legitimate focus of psychiatric research or treatment. Although valid prognosis is a goal of a phenomenological diagnosis, predictive validity is currently elusive for many categories.

Although it never died away completely, Kraepelin's descriptive approach was eclipsed by psychoanalysis during the middle decades of this century. Psychoanalytic diagnosis relies to a large extent upon theory and inference, postulating unconscious phenomena that cannot be measured reliably. Its observational base has been limited to individual patients seen over long periods in the unique situation of psychoanalysis and upon systematic observations of normal children. While certain psychoanalytic categorizations and ideas were accepted into the DSM, the manual explicitly repudiated psychoanalysis' theoretical base. Thus, it cannot be described as a reconciliation of the two traditions.

The main benefit of the DSM is that it **standardizes psychiatric diagnoses**, so that different people dealing with the same patient will use the same language to communicate about what they see. Agreement among multiple observers is measured statistically as reliability. Researchers and those who design treatment or reimbursement protocols require reliability to generalize findings or regulations from one population to another. While reliability is an important aspect of diagnosis, it is not a substitute for validity. A more valid classification might be one based on etiology. Such a scheme would not be purely phenomenological. One cause can generate different phenomena and similar phenomena may have differing causes. Thus, in an etiologic scheme, things that look similar might be placed in separate categories, while apparently different manifestations could be placed together, linked by a shared cause. An ideal scheme would be high in both reliability and validity, allowing those who use it to predict course of illness and treatment response. As a phenomenologic scheme, the DSM falls short of this standard.

Match the DSM axis in the numbered items with the **BEST** description of its domain from the following list.

(A) Psychiatric disorders related to underlying neurologic dysfunction.

(B) Psychiatric syndromes related to underlying neurologic or medical conditions.

(C) Clinical disorders, conditions that may be the focus of psychiatric attention.

(D) Physical or medical conditions causally related to a defined psychiatric disorder.

(E) Any physical or medical condition (causative of, resulting from, or unrelated to a defined psychiatric disorder).

(F) Personality disorders/habitual psychological defenses/mental retardation.

(G) Psychosexual developmental stage.

(H) Psychosocial/environmental problems that contribute to the development of a psychiatric disorder or may exacerbate it.

(I) Severity of recent personal events (current and in past year).

(J) Global assessment of function.

(K) Rating of severity of disorder on a scale of 1-5.

107. Axis I

108. Axis II

109. Axis III

110. Axis IV

111. Axis V

ANSWERS AND TUTORIAL ON ITEMS 107-111

The answers are: **107-C; 108-F; 109-E; 110-H; 111-J**. The Research Diagnostic Criteria (RDC), a detailed scheme for classifying the most serious and presumptively neurophysiologically based mental disorders for research purposes, provided a starting point for the modern DSMs. Reflecting this research heritage, disorders on the two primary axes are classified, whenever possible, in terms of symptoms that can be assessed reliably and behaviors that can be observed and quantified. However, the DSM is much broader and less rigorous than the RDC, being intended for clinical description, insurance reimbursement, many different kinds of research, and for communication between mental health professionals or with legal authorities. Thus, the DSM strives to capture the whole range of conditions seen and treated by psychiatrists, many of which do not involve underlying brain dysfunction. It has appeared in three versions over ten years, with DSM-III published in 1980, IIIR a few years later, and **DSM-IV** in 1995.

The clinical comprehensiveness of the DSM accounts for its apparently arbitrary qualities, for example, the placing of both major psychiatric syndromes and various life problems on **Axis I**, because either may be a focus of clinical attention, grounds for research, or grounds for insurance reimbursement. Thus, Axis I provides detailed descriptive criteria for conditions ranging from severe disorders like schizophrenia, for which research is gradually elucidating genetic, physiological and psychosocial mechanisms, to life issues sanctified by custom as appropriate for psychiatric attention. The latter ("v codes") include bereavement, problems in intimate relationships, career problems, and the like.

Axis II provides a system for classifying personality, a subject that was always of greater interest to psychoanalysis than to biological psychiatry. Axis II also includes mental retardation because this is considered, like personality, to be an enduring quality of a person, rather than a discrete disease or disorder. In the years between DSM-III and DSM-IV, clinical use of the system blurred the definition of Axis II somewhat. It is now legitimate to use Axis II to describe habitual psychological defenses, even in the absence of a definable personality disorder.

Axis III in DSM-IV includes any medical condition, not just conditions relevant to the person's Axis I condition (the DSM-III standard).

Axis IV was originally a numerical rating of current psychosocial stressors, but this proved to be unreliable. In DSM-IV, meaningful psychosocial events are merely listed and may include remote events, e.g., trauma, that may cause or exacerbate patients' presenting problems.

Axis V has evolved from a 1-5 rating of current function to the use of the Global Assessment Scale, which combines occupational, relational and psychological functioning in a single numerical rating on a scale ranging from 1 to 100.

Items 112-114

Choose the **BEST** response.

112. An interview designed to arrive at an appropriate DSM-IV diagnosis routinely covers all the following **EXCEPT**:

   (A) nature and course of symptomatology (present illness)
   (B) assessment of characteristic defenses
   (C) history of past psychiatric diagnoses and treatment
   (D) family history of psychiatric disorders, including substance abuse
   (E) mental status examination

113. Evaluation of a psychiatric patient should cover

   (A) history of important relationships, beginning with parents and siblings and including friends, colleagues, and intimate partners
   (B) beliefs and prejudices about psychiatric disorders and their treatment
   (C) school and work history
   (D) A and C only
   (E) A, B, and C

114. In an initial diagnostic interview, the clinician should always enquire about

   (A) dreams and fantasies
   (B) past and current medical problems
   (C) family medical history
   (D) A and C only
   (E) A, B, and C

ANSWERS AND TUTORIAL ON ITEMS 112-114

The answers are: **112-B; 113-E; 114-B**. The **initial psychiatric interview** has several purposes: to arrive at a phenomenological diagnosis; to develop understanding of the patient as a person with a unique history, a repertoire of defenses, recurrent areas of difficulty if present, and typical patterns of relating to others (psychodynamic formulation), and to identify factors that may enhance or impede treatment. A full interview requires investigation of present illness, past psychiatric diagnoses and treatment, family psychiatric history, medical history, developmental/social history and mental status examination. Different parts of the interview serve different purposes. The diagnosis of disorders on **Axis I** largely depends on symptomatology (present and in evolution over time), mental status, and current functional capacity. The social history identifies areas of impairment, which are core diagnostic criteria for most conditions. **Family psychiatric history** and response to prior treatment will tend to confirm or cast doubt on a diagnosis arrived at in this way. Medical history allows for the identification of Axis I disorders related to medical conditions.

The **assessment of defenses** is more important to arriving at a psychodynamic formulation, which will be based in part on the history of the person's patterns of relating to others, recurring areas of difficulty or conflict, and his or her mastery of age-appropriate developmental tasks. Some of this assessment requires the interviewer to draw inferences from both the facts of a person's history and from the way in which it is told. Patients' language, self-description, and attitude toward the interviewer provide clues to their characteristic defenses and core conflictual issues. At times, the developmental history and the interviewer's inferences will point to the diagnosis of a personality disorder on **Axis II**, but the definitions of these diagnoses exclude explicit references to defenses. Thus, the assessment of defenses is not a necessary part of DSM-IV based diagnosis, despite its relevance to constructing a psychodynamic formulation and fostering helpful clinician-patient interaction.

Eliciting patients' beliefs, preferences and prejudices about mental illness and psychiatric treatment is an important part of an initial interview, though not specific to the tasks of diagnosis or formulation. These elements are part of the assessment of factors that will likely enhance or impede treatment.

Exploration of **dreams and fantasies** is often a part of **psychodynamic psychotherapy**. Such exploration requires more free-flowing interaction than is possible in a structured diagnostic interview. Family medical history also has very little bearing on the diagnosis of current psychiatric disorders, though it may be relevant in other ways, for example, by opening up discussion of the person's experience dealing with a family member's chronic illness or death, or by uncovering fears for a person's own health. Past and current medical problems are highly relevant to diagnosis, since physical illnesses and prescribed medications can cause a variety of psychiatric syndromes. DSM-IV diagnosis requires specification of active medical conditions on **Axis III**.

Items 115-119

Choose the **BEST** response.

115. The mental status examination

    (A) Includes systematic observations of appearance, mood, affect, level of consciousness, speech, thought form, and thought content. May also involve screening tests of memory, concentration/attention, calculation, abstraction and judgment.
    (B) Incorporates parts of some scales from the Wechsler Adult Intelligence Scale (WAIS or IQ test), which provides norms for interpretation.
    (C) Exists in specialized forms, such as the Mini-Mental State Examination or Folstein test, for the detection of organic brain dysfunction.
    (D) All of the above
    (E) None of the above

116. All of the following categories of mental status are rated based on the interviewer's observations of the patient during history taking **EXCEPT**:

    (A) orientation
    (B) appearance
    (C) speech
    (D) thought form
    (E) level of consciousness

117. In recording mental status, all the following are moods of particular relevance to psychiatric disorders **EXCEPT**:

    (A) anxiety
    (B) euphoria
    (C) paranoia
    (D) sadness
    (E) anger

118. Typical disorders of thought form or process characteristic of psychosis include

    (A) circumstantiality
    (B) loosening of associations
    (C) tangentiality
    (D) A and C only
    (E) A, B, and C

119. In rating thought content, the examiner records evidence of

(A) delusions
(B) ideas of reference
(C) suicidal ideation
(D) A and C only
(E) A, B, and C

Items 120-123

Match the following tests to the intellectual functions they are **BEST** designed to measure. Answers may be used once, more than once, or not at all.

(A) Serial subtractions of 7 from 100 ("serial sevens")
(B) Digit span forwards and backwards
(C) Proverb interpretation
(D) Questions of general information
(E) Immediate repetition of three or four objects
(F) Repetition of objects after five minutes
(G) Giving name, date, place
(H) Following a series of commands

120. Orientation

121. Anterograde (short-term) memory

122. Registration

123. Abstraction

Items 124-128

Choose the **BEST** response.

124. Impairment of attention is revealed in patients' ability to

(A) perform serial sevens
(B) repeat three objects immediately after they are presented
(C) repeat digits forward and backwards
(D) A and C only
(E) A, B, and C

125. The term anterograde amnesia refers to inability to

    (A)   remember new information
    (B)   access information acquired previously
    (C)   access memories acquired under stressful emotional conditions
    (D)   A and C only
    (E)   None of the above

126. On the mental status examination, patients who complain of memory loss following electroconvulsive therapy will show

    (A)   loss of important, previously learned information (e.g., ability to practice one's profession)
    (B)   inability to remember events immediately before and in the first hours after treatment
    (C)   retrograde amnesia for the three or four days prior to treatment
    (D)   A and C only
    (E)   None of the above

127. The Mini-Mental State Examination differs from the standard mental status examination in

    (A)   allowing for orientation to be gradated rather than reported simply as intact or impaired
    (B)   including tests for language disorder as well as thought disorder
    (C)   including tests of sequencing and praxis
    (D)   A and C only
    (E)   A, B, and C

128. The Mini-Mental State Examination

    (A)   is a rapid screen for organic brain dysfunction
    (B)   is comprehensive in recording mental phenomena relevant to psychiatric populations
    (C)   can be used to follow patients over time as their mental status improves or deteriorates
    (D)   A and C only
    (E)   A, B, and C

ANSWERS AND TUTORIAL ON ITEMS 115-128

The answers are: **115-D; 116-A; 117-C; 118-E; 119-E; 120-G; 121-F; 122-E; 123-C; 124-E; 125-A; 126-B; 127-E; 128-D**. The **mental status examination** is a specialized portion of a psychiatric evaluation. Its purpose is to document the manifestations of disorder on which the clinician is basing his or her diagnosis. Clinicians also use it to screen for disorders other than the presenting one and to assess dimensions of illness (especially organic brain dysfunction and dangerousness) important across many conditions. The examiner first records observations of the patient's appearance, mood/affect, and thought form/thought content, as revealed in speech during the diagnostic interview. Observations in each of these domains are not random; rather they derive from descriptive models that specify the cardinal features of particular conditions. Thus, the examiner does not search for exact subtle words to capture the full range of the patient's mood or affect, but notes whether certain gross disruptions are present or absent. The moods of interest in psychiatric diagnosis are euphoria, sadness, anxiety, and anger (and related terms). Paranoia is considered a quality of thought rather than mood and is recorded under thought content.

Mental status findings do not by themselves confirm or rule out a particular **diagnosis**, but they do suggest the presence or absence of particular **syndromes**. Thus, **psychosis**, defined as a state in which inner mental experience pre-empts or distorts the appreciation of external reality, is not a disorder but a collection of symptoms that may be organized into an identifiable syndrome. Psychotic symptoms include mental status findings of abnormalities of perception (hallucinations), thought form, and thought content (delusions) (see Chapter VI). These occur in the course of a variety of disorders, including schizophrenia, mood disorders, delirium and dementia. In Item 118 (E) is correct because while **loosening of associations** is most commonly described in relation to mania, it may appear in any psychotic state. Loosening of associations occurs toward the more pathological end of a continuum of thought form abnormalities or **thought disorder.** Manifestations of thought disorder include blocking, circumstantiality, tangentiality, flight of ideas, loosening of associations, and incoherence or word salad.

Recording of **thought content** includes everything from the main themes in the self-description of a depressed outpatient to the delusions of one who is severely psychotic. It is a critical aspect of the mental status examination for several reasons. Firstly, it presents the world from the patient's point of view, an important place for the clinician to start if he or she means to establish rapport. The second crucial feature of recording thought content is that it reminds the clinician to screen every patient for suicidal, homicidal or assaultive thoughts and intentions (dangerousness). Sometimes patients fail to volunteer this information, which is, obviously, crucial to their care. Finally, certain disorders produce predictable abnormalities of thought content--mania engenders grandiosity, schizophrenia leads not only to delusions in general but to bizarre delusions or delusions of external influence (ideas of reference). Recording the presence or absence of these elements of mental status helps confirm or rule out diagnoses suggested by the patient's history.

The second part of a mental status examination involves screening for **neurologic impairment** (organicity). Clinicians tend to use a few questions drawn from subtests of standardized psychological test batteries, most commonly the Wechsler Adult Intelligence Scale

(WAIS). The cognitive functions screened include orientation, attention/concentration, ability to perform simple calculations, recall and recent memory, and ability to abstract. Assessment of long-term memory, ability to sequence information, vocabulary, judgment, and retention of learned information may be included. Often clinicians can rate these latter functions based on the person's ability to give an orderly history, without administering a specialized test.

The different mental status probes do not test specific functions in a clean or precise fashion. **Serial sevens**, for example, requires concentration but also the ability to perform simple calculations. Attention/concentration is a gateway function. Severe impairment in this area will cause patients to do poorly on almost every other mental status test. Milder attention problems will disrupt serial calculations, digit span, and registration of objects presented to test memory, but may leave the patient able to demonstrate abstraction, judgment, and retained information.

The classification of **memory** is an evolving field. Currently, scholars differentiate anterograde memory (ability to learn new information) from retrograde memory (ability to access previously acquired information). Other classifications distinguish registration, retention, and recall or immediate, short-term (recent) and long-term (remote, past) memory. No system corresponds exactly to another. Immediate memory, or registration, involves taking in information as it is presented. Short-term memory connotes memories retained for several minutes up to twenty four hours. Remote or long-term memory or recall covers all other memory, sometimes subclassified into memories of the past few months (recent past memory) and older memories.

These distinctions are meaningful because different disorders may spare one memory function while damaging another. Thus, patients in a postictal state (including following electroconvulsive therapy) may have brief retrograde amnesia for immediately preceding events and a longer anterograde amnesia for the events following the seizure. Delirium, which affects level of consciousness and attention, will typically impair both registration and retention/short-term memory. In alcohol-induced persistent amnestic disorder (Korsakoff's syndrome), registration and long-term memory are relatively preserved, while short-term memory is severely impaired. Anterograde and short-term memory are affected first in dementia of the Alzheimer's type, with retrograde/long-term memory deteriorating in later stages of the illness.

The **Mini-Mental State Examination** (MMSE) is a standardized version of the neurological screening portion of a clinical mental status examination. It involves, first, asking the patient to give up to ten aspects of orientation in time and place. The next questions assess concentration, registration and short-term memory (recall). The examiner then tests the language functions of naming, repetition, reading, writing, copying, and following a three stage command. The test has been standardized in normal, psychiatrically, and neurologically ill populations. It is highly sensitive to cognitive impairment and can differentiate impairment from psychiatric and neurologic (structural brain) processes relatively well. Because the MMSE is quantitative, clinicians use it to follow patients as they improve or deteriorate with treatment. However, the MMSE does not screen for many salient psychiatric variables (suicidality, psychosis, mood, etc.) and so is not comprehensive.

Items 129-132

Each of the following mental status examinations in the items below points to a particular psychiatric syndrome. Match the number of the case to the **MOST** appropriate diagnostic description from answers below. Answers may be used only once or not at all.

(A)   Delirium
(B)   Amnestic disorder (Korsakoff's psychosis)
(C)   Pseudodementia
(D)   Generalized Anxiety
(E)   Depression
(F)   Mania
(G)   Schizophreniform psychosis
(H)   Delusional disorder

129.   Case I

Appearance: Disheveled 52-year-old woman with excess makeup, tight fitting clothes and elaborate manicure, with some broken nails
Level of consciousness: Alert
Mood: Euphoric, irritable
Affect: Cheerful, inappropriate at times (giggles describing loss)
Speech: Pressured, emphatic
Thought form: Flight of ideas without loose associations; circumstantiality
Thought content: Grandiose plans to start her own business, take over the hospital; content is quite fluid and she rationalizes extensively when challenged; some assaultive thoughts but not homicidal or suicidal. No hallucinations admitted. Fleeting paranoid ideas that she does not cling to. No ideas of reference.
Formal testing: Oriented X 2.5 (off by one day on date); 3/3 objects at five minutes, remote memory apparently normal except some confusion in sequencing; Can name presidents backward to Carter (omitting Ford); Serial sevens done rapidly with three errors; digit span six forward, four backward; Continuous performance testing: no errors; **Proverbs**: Abstract, personalized; Formal judgment: would mail a stamped letter, knows why criminals are locked up, but history suggests personal judgment impaired (spent $600 on winter clothes in July; keeps calling her ex-husband, despite restraining order)

130. Case II

Appearance: Unshaven young man in tattered clothing
Level of consciousness: Alert
Mood: Mildly depressed
Affect: Flat
Speech: Long latency in response to questions, laconic
Thought form: Circumstantial, tangential, some odd associations
Thought content: Delusional; believes that world is color coded and that he has to figure out who is safe and who is evil based on what they wear; ideas of reference: gets special messages from the television and from what he reads, is sure people are talking about him when around strangers; auditory hallucinations of voices commenting on his behavior; no admitted suicidal ideation (SI); some desire to mutilate self
Formal testing: Oriented X 3; recalls 3/3 objects at five minutes; remote memory grossly intact; categories concrete; proverbs, concrete ("The glass will break.") Serial sevens done slowly with one error. Seven digits forward, five in reverse. Calculations: Knows there are 20 nickels in a dollar and that sixty nickels equal three dollars. Formal judgment: Would leave a letter in the street; Knows why criminals are locked up. By history, impaired judgment (acts in ways based on his delusions)

131. Case III

Appearance: 45-year-old woman, neatly dressed, looks sad, inexpressive
Level of consciousness: Alert
Mood: Depressed, subdued
Affect: Sad, overtly tearful at times
Speech: Normal, though some hesitancy around painful topics
Thought form: Unremarkable
Thought content: Themes of inadequacy, hopelessness, worry, including worry about her health. Passive suicidal ideation without plan or intent; No hallucinations or delusions or ideas of reference
Formal testing: Oriented X 3, 3/3 objects at five minutes, 7 digits forward, 5 backward, proverbs and categories abstract, serial sevens done slowly with no errors; Gives up reciting presidents after Reagan; calculations normal; formal judgment normal; personal judgment: has some insight into own condition.

132. Case IV

Appearance: 60 yr old man dressed in hospital pajamas
Level of consciousness: Alert
Mood: Euthymic
Affect: Cheerful
Speech: Fluent, some syntactical errors (possibly consistent with level of education); regional accent
Thought form: Circumstantial, loses the thread of questions
Thought content: Wants to go home, live independently; no insight into problems that caused family to bring him in to hospital (poor self-care, including nutrition); No hallucinations, delusions or ideas of reference; Not homicidal or suicidal.
Formal testing: Oriented to name, place but not date. 3/3 objects immediately; O/3 objects at five minutes, can't recall what he had for breakfast. Unable to do digit span. Spells world forward but not backward. Loses the task of serial sevens after two steps. Simple calculations normal. Long-term memory grossly normal--knows his birthday, where he lived growing up, dates of military service, names of family members; categories--concrete; proverbs: refuses; formal judgment normal (would mail a letter, knows why criminals are locked up)

ANSWERS AND TUTORIAL ON ITEMS 129-132

The answers are: **129-F; 130-G; 131-E; 132-B. Case I** is a classic description of **mania** without clear evidence of psychosis. Thus, the patient is euphoric, pressured, and grandiose. Her disorganized appearance is consistent with her mild cognitive impairments (errors on serial sevens, slight disorientation, slightly reduced digit span). These are consistent with lack of attention/concentration or lack of motivation to respond accurately but not with severe brain dysfunction. The difference between her judgment as measured with a standardized question and as revealed in her history is typical in mania, where patients' behavior is often more disordered than their language and self-presentation would lead one to expect.

    Case II illustrates a **schizophreniform psychosis** in which cognitive functions are relatively intact, despite significant impairment in thought form, content, and mood.

    Case III describes **depression**, in which mood is more disordered than thought.

    Case IV is a realistic illustration of **Korsakoff's syndrome**, most typically a sequela of thiamine deficiency in chronic alcoholics. Although short-term memory loss is the most striking aspect of this disorder, patients typically have mild impairment in other cognitive functions (e.g., disorientation in time, inability to remember a task long enough to complete it). Learned or rote material, which is tested by judgment questions, will be intact. In the setting of Korsakoff's syndrome, such questions do not test real world judgement very well. In daily life the ability to exercise good judgment requires being able to relate present circumstances to remembered ones. Patients who cannot remember recent experience or the nature of their impairments cannot take these factors into account when making decisions.

Items 133-140

The following items pertain to the epidemiology of suicide.

Choose the **BEST** response.

133. Choose from the following, the most accurate rank ordering of suicide risk factors (highest to lowest)

    (A)   prior suicide attempts; declining physical health; age greater than 45 (men), 55 (women); alcohol dependence; recent loss or separation; single, widowed or divorced

    (B)   recent loss or separation; single, widowed or divorced; alcohol dependence; declining physical health; age over 45 (men), 55 (women); prior suicide attempts

    (C)   age over 45 (men), 55 (women); alcohol dependence; prior suicide attempts; recent loss or separation; declining physical health; single, widowed or divorced

    (D)   alcohol dependence; age over 45 (men), 55 (women); prior suicide attempts; declining physical health; recent loss or separation; single, widowed or divorced

    (E)   declining physical health; recent loss or separation; alcohol dependence; age greater than 45 (men), 55 (women); prior suicide attempts; single, widowed or divorced.

134. Factors that lower suicide risk include

    (A)   stable employment
    (B)   female gender
    (C)   choice of nonviolent methods
    (D)   A and C only
    (E)   A, B and C

135. Among medical specialties, the one with the highest suicide rate is

    (A)   general practice
    (B)   anesthesiology
    (C)   ophthalmology
    (D)   psychiatry
    (E)   internal medicine

136. The rate of suicide among women physicians

    (A)   Is roughly three times that of white women of comparable ages.
    (B)   Shows an excess compared to controls, while the rate among male physicians is similar to that of controls.
    (C)   May in part reflect an unusually high risk for mood disorders among all women physicians.
    (D)   All of the above
    (E)   None of the above

137. A person with a history of several prior failed suicide attempts or gestures

    (A)   Is at less risk for suicide than a never-attempter.
    (B)   Has suicide risk equal to that of a never-attempter.
    (C)   Has a greater risk of suicide than a never-attempter.
    (D)   Has a greater risk of suicide than a never attempter only if a prior attempt failed accidentally.

138. Each of the following major psychiatric diagnoses has been associated with increased risk for suicide **EXCEPT**:

    (A)   depression
    (B)   schizophrenia
    (C)   substance dependence
    (D)   obsessive-compulsive disorder
    (E)   borderline personality disorder

139. The rate of completed suicide in mood disorder is

    (A)   2-8%
    (B)   10-15%
    (C)   15-20%
    (D)   20-25%
    (E)   > 25%

140. Across diagnostic categories, the biological marker most clearly associated with completed suicide by violent means is

    (A)   decreased norepinephrine in the locus ceruleus
    (B)   decreased serotonin metabolite (5-HIAA) in the cerebrospinal fluid
    (C)   increased dopamine metabolites (HVA, MHPG) in urine
    (D)   decreased dopamine metabolites (HVA, MHPG) in urine

ANSWERS AND TUTORIAL ON ITEMS 133-140

The answers are: **133-C; 134-E; 135-D; 136-E; 137-D; 138-D; 139-B; 140-B. Suicide**, the deliberate infliction of death on the self, was the first psychiatric problem to be studied epidemiologically and sociologically. This academic tradition has created a rich literature on variables associated with suicide attempts and completed suicide in large scale, retrospective, population based studies. These variables are called **risk factors**. Recognition of the presence of risk factors in individual patients is part of the evaluation of psychiatric patients. However, suicide is a rare event, even in very high risk populations. Counting up risk factors does not permit accurate prediction of suicide (or safety) in any particular case.

Despite the inherent unpredictability of suicide, all physicians should know that **advancing age, male sex, substance abuse, depression, single status, recent losses**, and **poor physical health** are the variables that account for the greatest percentage of the variance in studies of suicide. Older, depressed, single, alcoholic men in poor health should be assessed carefully, especially if they have sustained a recent loss. As a group, they tend to be noncompliant and difficult to treat, so that physicians must make a conscious effort to push for active intervention when such patients describe suicidal thoughts, especially if they have made prior attempts.

In assessing the suicidal patient, mitigating factors are as important as exacerbating ones. The nature of a person's plans--choice of unavailable or nonviolent methods, the high probability of rescue, the presence of strongly held beliefs against suicide--as well as the absence of demographic risk factors are protective to some degree. Being currently married with children lowers risk, though previously married people have higher rates than those who have never married. Regardless of protective factors, someone with suicidal plans is at greater risk that someone with passive ideation only.

Among psychiatric disorders, **depression**, which has a 15% mortality from suicide, confers the highest risk. However, suicide is a significant risk in many other disorders. Suicidal ideation is not a core criterion for **schizophrenia**, for example, yet the illness carries a 10% mortality from suicide. Any psychotic patient should be queried about suicidal ideation and behavior, although suicide in this population tends to more impulsive (that is, less often preceded by expressed plans or intent) than it is in depression. Obsessive-compulsive disorder, by itself, is not known to increase suicide risk. Patients with **borderline personality disorder** often make suicide attempts or are self-mutilating. Contrary to some popular myths, **prior attempts** are predictors of suicide, not signs that people do not intend really to kill themselves.

Suicide risk varies among physicians. In the U.S., male physicians do not have higher rates than males in the general population, perhaps because the rate among males in this country is so high. In Great Britain and Scandinavia, however, male physicians' risk is 2 to 3 times higher than that of the population. Women physicians in all countries are at higher risk than women in the general population, possibly because they also have a higher lifetime risk of mood disorders. While particular specialties, especially psychiatry, ophthalmology and anesthesiology, have higher suicide rates than others, the most important predictive variable among physicians remains the presence of a mood disorder or substance abuse. Other professional groups associated with increased risk include musicians, dentists, law enforcement personnel, lawyers, and insurance agents.

Many studies have found decreased **5-HIAA** in the CSF of suicidal (and violent) patients. This fact points to a common dysregulation of serotonin activity that cuts across diagnostic categories associated with impulsivity and violence. This test is not used clinically. It is invasive, technically difficult, and the range of values overlaps between violent subjects and controls.

Items 141-145

The following items pertain to the clinical assessment of suicide. Match the **MOST** appropriate intervention in the answers with the case vignette in the items below. Answers (interventions) may be used once, more than once, or not at all.

Interventions:

(A) Admit to hospital voluntarily.

(B) Offer voluntary hospitalization, but commit to hospital if patient refuses.

(C) Comfort and reassure; send home with instructions to avoid drugs and alcohol.

(D) Reassure the patient and send home after arranging for someone trustworthy to provide supervision until the first outpatient mental health visit.

(E) Admit to hospital if no reliable person can be found to stay with patient until outpatient treatment can be arranged.

(F) Refer to a physician who will help the patient commit suicide.

141. Case I: A 24-year-old woman who has just broken up with her boyfriend is brought to the emergency room by her roommate after taking an overdose of sleeping pills and alcohol. The door was unlocked and the patient was found lying in the living room. She reports, and her roommate confirms, that she is normally a social drinker. She admits to having made an overdose attempt under similar circumstances in high school. She says she "just didn't care about ever waking up" when she took the pills. She now feels embarrassed and says she was overreacting and won't try again.

142. Case II: A 22-year-old man who works as a stock clerk comes to the emergency room because of increasing thoughts of hanging himself. In the prior year, he was diagnosed as having schizoaffective disorder, after two separate brief hospitalizations for psychotic episodes. He has taken his medications erratically since discharge, complaining that he can't tolerate the fatigue and the weight gain. He has had some return of paranoid thoughts and auditory hallucinations. He drinks fairly heavily on weekends, as he did prior to hospitalization. He was unable to return to school following his hospitalization.

He has had to return to live with his mother, who, he feels, is constantly on his case about not having a better job.

143. Case III: A 60-year-old widow, mother of three grown children, with a history of hypertension and a prior left hemisphere stroke with residual weakness of the right leg, comes to the emergency room with a superficial cut on her wrist. She does not recall deciding she wanted to kill herself. "I had the knife in my hand to slice onions, and suddenly I cut on my wrist." The patient admits to feeling more sad recently, as she often feels around the anniversary of her husband's death. She also reports that she has been depressed since her stroke, with fragmented sleep, irritability, tearfulness and poor appetite. She does not drink and her only medication is clonidine for her blood pressure. In general, she cooperates with medical treatment, and she is glad to be told that her depression might be treatable.

144. Case IV: A 43-year-old, twice divorced man with a five year cocaine habit comes in asking for treatment. He has had intense suicidal ideation for the past two weeks, with a plan to jump from a nearby bridge. He also describes such depressive symptoms as fatigue, weight gain, sluggishness and self-loathing. He has abstained from cocaine for two weeks. When using, he drank about six beers per day. He has cut down to one per day, but he did drink himself into a state of unconsciousness over the prior weekend, after standing at the edge of a bridge for an hour, trying to decide whether or not to jump. His friends are all drug users and he is in danger of losing his job because of absenteeism. He cannot contract for safety if he goes home.

145. Case V: A 75-year-old married man with advanced prostate cancer requests assistance in committing suicide. He feels his life is no longer worth living, and he doesn't want to use up his wife's inheritance. He has considerable pain from bone metastases, and he says the pain causes much sleeplessness. His oncologist says he could live a year or more. He has been taking large amounts non-narcotic painkillers, which upset his stomach but have not adequately controlled the pain.

ANSWERS AND TUTORIAL ON ITEMS 141-145

The answers are: **141-D; 142-B; 143-E; 144-B; 145-D**. Each of these cases requires clinical judgment. However, **case I** (D) probably does not require hospitalization. Her suicide attempt was made with high probability of rescue, she was ambivalent at the time, she professes no ongoing suicidal intent, and there are people around to watch her. One of the immediate triggers of her suicidal behavior, alcohol, has presumably washed out of her system, and by history she should be able to follow instructions to avoid it. However, she has made a prior attempt, suggesting some longstanding difficulties handling loss and separation. This is grounds for outpatient mental health treatment, which should be strongly urged.

Case II (B), by contrast, has many aspects that prompt hospitalization. Psychiatric patients who commit suicide are often much younger than the age of highest risk in the general population. People recently diagnosed with a major psychotic disorder are at increased risk at the first year after diagnosis, after which the risk falls again, until it rises with age and chronicity. Recent discharge from the hospital, loss of functional capacity, and living in an environment where the patient faces criticism, inflated expectations, and lack of acceptance of illness (high **expressed emotion** or EE) are also risk factors. Finally, this patient's plan is potentially lethal, he uses alcohol unwisely, and he finds the side-effects of his treatment to be disabling. Increased compliance with outpatient treatment is unlikely unless he spends time in an environment where he is restabilized on medication, persuaded to forego alcohol, and participates in educational, emotion-lowering exercises with his mother. The presence of psychosis further suggests the use of involuntary commitment or certification, although it does not automatically justify such a step.

Case III (E) illustrates the risk of impulsive, self-destructive behavior in people with organic brain disorders. Depression is a common, undertreated sequela of stroke, especially strokes involving the left hemisphere. The lack of prior planning is not a protective factor in this case, since frontal lobe damage from the stroke or from multiple small infarcts related to hypertension may impair the capacity to plan. Mitigating against hospitalization, the patient seems to have no clear suicidal intent even after having hurt herself. Her method, though invasive, was of low lethality. Her antihypertensive medication is not particularly associated with depression, she avoids alcohol, and she seems likely to comply with outpatient treatment. Hospitalization would be indicated only if this patient could not be supervised at home. There is no reason to suspect that her social network would be unsupportive. Early follow up, with prescription of adequate doses of antidepressant medication, would probably be sufficient treatment. She might also be considered for partial hospitalization, again, supposing someone could be with her at night.

Case IV (B) should be hospitalized. Although his drug abuse raises the possibility that he is manipulating to escape his current environment, intense depression is a physiological manifestation of cocaine abstinence. His recent high level of alcohol use, which is common in cocaine users, is enough to further depress him, and he has not had even a month of full abstinence, the time required for this effect to improve. His method is of high lethality, he faces a serious potential loss with the situation on his job, and his coping skills (increasing alcohol use) are highly dysfunctional. His social network, moreover, is thin and unreliable. The common crisis intervention technique of contracting for safety (promising to call or return if suicidality worsens) helps physicians decide in borderline cases whether to admit a patient to the hospital or not. Although refusal to make a contract may be a sign of manipulativeness, previously unknown patients should be taken at face value if they are unable to make such promises. The use of commitment or certification if the patient refuses voluntary treatment is controversial in a case where the person is cognitively intact. However, depression following cocaine withdrawal can be severe enough to impair competence and judgment by making patients hopeless about treatment. Commitment or certification, with early judicial review, would be defensible in this case.

In **Case V** (D), the request for assisted suicide is best viewed as a call for help. The legal status of assisted suicide is highly uncertain; even referral to another practitioner would be unethical. More importantly, the vast majority of patients who request assisted suicide, even if terminally ill, change their minds after adequate treatment for depression and pain. A combination of opiates, antidepressants, possibly palliative radiation, and self-hypnosis could be very helpful to this patient. Couples or family meetings to discuss the best use of common resources are also indicated. These represent better coping than a unilateral decision on the part of the patient to try to protect his wife's interests. Unless the patient seems about to take matters into his or her own hands if the request is refused, hospitalization is not indicated. People with chronic conditions should be maintained in their usual home environments as much as possible. This patient is not alone, does not drink, and has a treatable illness--depression--as well as an untreatable one. Thus, answer D is correct.

CHAPTER IV
DISORDERS OF CHILDHOOD

Items 146-149

Choose the **BEST** response.

146. All of the following statements regarding mental retardation (MR) are **TRUE EXCEPT**:

    (A)   diagnosed before age 18
    (B)   characterized by low intelligence and impairment in social functioning
    (C)   most cases are caused by inborn errors of metabolism
    (D)   defined as IQ below 70
    (E)   prevalence is the general population is about 1%

147. All of the following are known causes of mental retardation **EXCEPT**:

    (A)   fragile X syndrome
    (B)   Down's syndrome (trisomy 21)
    (C)   hypothyroidism
    (D)   phenylketonuria
    (E)   tuberous sclerosis

148. Intelligence quotient (IQ) in children is **BEST** defined as

    (A)   chronological age X mental age ÷ 100
    (B)   mental age ÷ chronological age X 100
    (C)   one standard deviation below the mean
    (D)   chronological age ÷ mental age X 100
    (E)   total score on Wechsler Intelligence Scale for Children-Revised (WISC-R)

149. Which of the following statements regarding the epidemiology of mental retardation is **TRUE?**

    (A)   It is equally distributed among males and females.
    (B)   All forms are more common in lower socioeconomic classes.
    (C)   Down's syndrome is the most common genetic cause.
    (D)   In most cases of severe MR, the etiology is unknown.
    (E)   Rarely observed in children suffering from fetal alcohol syndrome.

ANSWERS AND TUTORIAL ON ITEMS 146-149

The answers are: **146-C; 147-E; 148-B; 149-C. Mental retardation** (MR) is relatively common in the general population. Its prevalence is about 1-2%. While milder cases of MR are more common in the lower socioeconomic classes, cases of moderate and severe MR are equally distributed in the population. For the majority of **severe** cases, MR stems from genetic, infectious, nutritional, metabolic, toxic, or traumatic causes. The etiology in most cases of **mild** MR is unknown. There is a 2:1 M:F sex ratio for MR.

The diagnosis of MR requires demonstration of a subnormal IQ as determined by standardized testing, such as the **Wechsler Intelligence Scale for Children-Revised** (WISC-R) together with impairment in adaptive social functioning. It has to be diagnosed prior to age 18 and in most cases is evident quite early in childhood. **Intelligence quotient** (IQ) is defined as mental age (obtained by psychological testing) ÷ chronological age X 100. An IQ of 70 is chosen as the arbitrary cutoff point for MR, since it falls two standard deviations below the population mean.

The most common cause of MR is **fetal alcohol syndrome**. The most common genetic cause of MR is **Down's syndrome**. Other less common genetic causes include fragile X syndrome, cri du chat syndrome, and Prader-Willi syndrome. Inborn errors of metabolism leading to MR include Tay-Sachs disease and phenylketonuria. Untreated infantile hypothyroidism, maternal exposure to rubella virus, perinatal and postnatal trauma, and CNS infections can also lead to MR. **Tuberous sclerosis** is a neurocutaneous syndrome characterized by CNS calcifications, skin eruptions, and seizures. It is not known to cause MR.

The parents of a 4-year-old boy bring him in for evaluation. Being their second child, he seemed consistently slower in development compared to his older sister. At age three, he spoke only a few words and did not seem to attempt to form sentences. He was also late to sit, crawl, and walk. Once having learned to carry out gross motor tasks, he remained quite clumsy. To date, he has not been toilet trained. While slow to develop, he is, nonetheless, quite attached to his parents and plays well with other children. For a while, the parents attributed his slowness to the fact that "boys develop more slowly than girls" but they are becoming increasingly concerned about their son's lack of progress.

Choose the **BEST** response.

150.   As an evaluating physician, you should

    (A)   Reassure the parents. It is normal for boys to lag in development.
    (B)   Ask the parents to bring the sister for comparative assessment.
    (C)   Refer the parents to a child psychiatrist with the suspicion of autism.
    (D)   Obtain detailed family, antenatal, perinatal, and postnatal history. Perform thorough physical and neurological examinations.
    (E)   Refer the child to a therapeutic nursery.

151.   Which of the following tests would be appropriate in evaluating this youngster?

    (A)   hearing and speech assessment
    (B)   EEG and MRI
    (C)   karyotype analysis
    (D)   psychological testing
    (E)   All of the above

152.   After a review of all tests and examinations, you diagnose the boy with mental retardation. What is the expected course of his condition?

    (A)   His functioning will improve with age.
    (B)   He will eventually catch up with his peers in current developmental delays.
    (C)   He will slowly deteriorate and eventually require institutionalization.
    (D)   The course of this condition is unpredictable.
    (E)   The course largely depends on the type and severity of mental retardation.

153. The treatment of children with MR should include

   (A) Correction of all treatable causes such as hypothyroidism, infections, and metabolic deficiencies.
   (B) Behavioral therapy and social skills training.
   (C) Support for the family.
   (D) Appropriate educational assessment and placement.
   (E) All of the above

ANSWERS AND TUTORIAL ON ITEMS 150-153

The answers are: **150-D; 151-E; 152-E; 153-E.** The clinical presentation of **mental retardation** (MR) takes place prior to age 18. In most cases, low intellectual functioning is evident early in childhood, and, certainly, by school age. In young children, intelligence is closely linked to the development of language. Additionally, timely achievement of developmental milestones roughly corresponds to maturity of the CNS.

In the clinical vignette, the boy demonstrates difficulties in a number of areas, specifically language development, motor skills, and social training. His inability to be toilet trained speaks to both the immaturity of his CNS and lack of social learning. While girls tend, on the average, to develop language skills a few months earlier than boys, and may be toilet trained sooner, they are not necessarily quicker to develop motor skills. What differentiates MR from **autism** is the clear presence of attachment and social reciprocity in this boy. Referral to either a child psychiatrist or a therapeutic nursery is premature. Careful physical and neurological examination is warranted because they may reveal the causes of developmental delays which are potentially treatable. Likewise, pre-, peri-, and postnatal history may bring to light treatable causes of MR or at least establish etiology.

In the evaluation of MR, chromosomal analysis may uncover underlying genetic defects. Seizures and nonspecific CNS pathology are common in MR, therefore an EEG and MRI are indicated. Since language development is dependent on intact hearing, speech and hearing assessment is warranted. Psychological testing will further define neuropsychological deficits and determine IQ.

The course of the condition largely depends on the extent of the MR. In severe cases, the course can be degenerative and lead to death at an early age. In milder cases, expected development occurs, only at a slower pace. The child's ability to adjust to the demands of everyday life is related to the severity of the retardation, the availability of rehabilitation services, and appropriate social skills training.

Choose the **BEST** response.

154. Autistic disorder is thought to be due to

    (A)   a chromosomal numerical anomaly
    (B)   a perinatal viral infection, resulting in subclinical encephalitis
    (C)   a genetic anomaly of unknown origin
    (D)   a metabolic anomaly of unknown origin
    (E)   a slow viral infection, similar to Creutzfeldt-Jakob disease

155. All of the following are necessary diagnostic criteria for autism according to the DSM-IV **EXCEPT**:

    (A)   onset after 36 months
    (B)   failure to develop age appropriate peer relationships
    (C)   lack of social reciprocity
    (D)   stereotyped and repetitive use of language
    (E)   delay in or total lack of development of spoken language

156. Which of the following is **TRUE** regarding autism?

    (A)   male:female ratio is 4:1
    (B)   prevalence is 1/1,000
    (C)   the disorder is familial
    (D)   A and C only
    (E)   A, B, and C

157. Which of the following differentiate autism from mental retardation?

    (A)   delays in language development
    (B)   lack of social reciprocity
    (C)   low intellectual functioning
    (D)   higher incidence of seizures
    (E)   male predominance

158. Which of the following behaviors is **RARELY** present in autism?

    (A)   self-mutilation
    (B)   stereotyped movements
    (C)   auditory hallucinations
    (D)   rigid adherence to nonfunctional routines
    (E)   lack of eye contact

159. All of the following confer good prognosis in autistic disorder **EXCEPT**:

  (A)   normal to high IQ
  (B)   development of language
  (C)   development of social skills
  (D)   presence of repetitive movements

ANSWERS AND TUTORIAL ON ITEMS 154-159

The answers are: **154-C; 155-A; 156-E; 157-B; 158-C; 159-D**. **Autism** is one of the pervasive developmental disorders. It presents early in childhood and is readily apparent by age 3. It is defined by impairment in three domains: social interactions, communication, and the development of symbolic play. The impairment in social interactions is evident in lack of attachment behavior, desire to share one's experiences with others, development of peer relationships, social reciprocity, and nonverbal behaviors. Language development is frequently delayed and may never take place. The language of children who eventually learn to talk is characterized by idiosyncrasies, inability to initiate reciprocal communications, and linguistic stereotypies. Imaginative play is severely impaired. Instead, there is a preponderance of repetitive motions, and preoccupation in one area of interest, such as scheduling or counting. Additionally, forms of self-mutilation such as head banging or hand biting are common. Comorbid **seizure disorders** are also common in people with autism.

The prevalence of autism is on the order of 1/1,000. It has a male:female ratio of 4:1. The etiology of autism is unclear but there is a familial aggregation of cases of autism. The concordance rate for monozygotic twins is significantly higher than that for dizygotic twins. The specific mode of genetic transmission has not been identified. Of interest is a consistent neuroanatomic finding of **ventricular enlargement** in the brains of autistic children. Autism shares this finding with schizophrenia.

The clinical course of autism is **chronic**. Most abnormalities persist into adulthood, making education and independent living an unusual outcome in most cases. Factors that confer a better prognosis include normal or near normal intelligence, functional language acquisition, and relative sparing of social dysfunction.

Items 160-167

Match the clinical vignette in the items below with the **MOST** appropriate diagnosis in the list of answers. Answers may be used once, more than once, or not at all.

     (A)   Autism
     (B)   Mental retardation
     (C)   Attention-deficit/hyperactivity disorder
     (D)   Schizophrenia, childhood onset
     (E)   Reading disorder
     (F)   Conduct disorder
     (G)   Tourette's disorder
     (H)   Separation anxiety disorder
     (I)   Enuresis

160.   Bill is six years old. He has a few friends and plays well with his peers. Ever since the start of school, though, he has been experiencing difficulties in learning the alphabet and learning to spell and read. He does not appear slow in other areas, but is quite distraught over his difficulties, and, of late, refuses to play with other boys.

161.   Suzie has always been a somewhat withdrawn child. With age, she has grown more aloof and uninterested in friends and normal childhood games. She spends much time in her room, fixated on dinosaurs, and plays only with dinosaur toys. Sometimes, she talks to herself or responds to somebody not obviously present. She speaks of hearing distant roars of dinosaurs, who give her special messages.

162.   John is five years old. He speaks incomprehensibly in monosyllables. His speech is rarely directed to somebody, and he appears to speak to himself. He spends his free time sitting in the corner of the room, rocking, and gets quite upset if disturbed from that activity. When addressed, he avoids eye contact and does not return a smile.

163.   Tony is a six-year-old boy brought in for evaluation of poor school performance and peer relationships. He is fidgety, shifts his attention rapidly, and seem unable to sit still. Among the problems reported are incomplete assignments and frequent fights in school.

164.   Janet is five years old. Her mother notes that while playing with other children on the playground, Janet frequently does not wait her turn and seems to be unable to follow the rules of the game. Likewise, she does not play well alone. Janet does not complete even simple tasks and seems to be constantly "on the go". Janet's mother wonders if Janet understands what is asked of her.

165.   Fred is brought in for an evaluation by his parents at the insistence of the school counselor. Fred, who is twelve now, has always been "a problem kid". His school work

has been barely passable. While he does have a group of friends, they, too, always seem to be in trouble. He easily gets into fights, is inconsiderate of others, and skips school frequently. Recently, he and his buddies attracted the attention of the police for smoking marijuana.

166.   Annie is brought in by her mother because of recent refusal to attend school. For the past two months following a bad case of the flu, Annie has complained of persistent stomach ache. She is afraid to go to school for fear of getting ill in class. She is more clingy than usual. Of late, she worries that her mother may not be there when she returns home from school.

167.   Elliot is embarrassed to attend school. He recently noticed that periodically he makes strange barking and grunting sounds. Initially, he thought he was just clearing his throat, but he has become increasingly aware of having little or no control over these noises. Upon examination, he exhibits occasional facial grimacing and eye blinking.

ANSWERS AND TUTORIAL ON ITEMS 160-167

The answers are: **160-E; 161-D; 162-A; 163-C; 164-C; 165-F; 166-H; 167-G**. In the first vignette, the most likely diagnosis is **reading disorder**. Bill is experiencing difficulties only in the area of reading. There is no evidence of impairment in other academic domains or areas of function, which might suggest MR. Additionally, Bill has demonstrated the ability to form friendships and to engage in social interactions, which effectively rules out autism. His recent refusal to play with peers is not unusual for a child who is having any academic difficulty. Since school performance becomes a major contributor to self-esteem in the latency-age child, problems in this area are often accompanied by disruption of peer relationships.

Suzie's withdrawal and social isolation are ominous symptoms. In the histories of many children and adolescents who later develop schizophrenia, social withdrawal predominates in the prodromal stage of the illness. Among the diagnostic possibilities are autism, especially in view of the lack of interpersonal relationships and presence of intense preoccupation with a single theme (dinosaurs). Also, depression must be considered. What makes Suzie's condition suggestive of **schizophrenia of childhood onset**, is the presence of auditory hallucinations, as evidenced by her talking to herself, responding to internal stimuli, and having ideas of reference (special messages, intended only for her). While a number of these elements may be present in normal fantasy play, isolation and withdrawal are pathologic. Likewise, auditory hallucinations may be found in both autism and MR, but they are rare and not prominent.

John demonstrates profound deficits in linguistic development suggestive of **autism**. Not only has he not formed comprehensible language by age five, his ability to use language as a tool of social communication is impaired as well. His isolation and stereotyped, repetitive activity in conjunction with lack of reciprocity in social cuing is most consistent with the diagnosis of autism.

Tony presents with symptoms of overactivity and inattention. There are elements of social difficulties and academic problems. The picture is most consistent with the diagnosis of **attention-deficit/hyperactivity disorder** (ADHD). While Tony's fights in school ought to raise, at least, a consideration of conduct disorder, there is not enough evidence to suggest that he meets criteria for this disorder. Moreover, ADHD and conduct disorder are frequently comorbid conditions. Statistically, one third of children with ADHD may go on to develop a conduct disorder. Fights, difficulties with peers, and impulsivity are characteristics shared by both conditions. The case of Janet is similar. In younger children, impulsivity and hyperactivity are seen in the inability to take turns, especially on the playground. While Janet's mother is concerned with Janet's understanding, Janet's problem is not a lack of intelligence, but an impairment in attention.

Fred demonstrates a number of symptoms indicative of serious difficulties. In addition to poor academic performance, he presents with behavioral problems of an antisocial type. His persistent fighting, disregard for others, truancy, and use of illicit drugs all are consistent with the diagnosis of **conduct disorder**. While he seems to have peer relationships, their nature is an affiliation with a gang. The natural outcome of conduct disorder in childhood is the development of **antisocial personality disorder** in adulthood.

Annie presents with typical **separation anxiety disorder**. While separation anxiety itself is a normal aspect of growth and development, and, to a degree, persists into adulthood, separation anxiety disorder is defined by impairment in social and occupational functioning, as well as by duration of disturbance for at least four weeks. It is not unusual for the disorder to be precipitated by a prolonged illness of either the child or the parent, or preceded by family stress. Intense closeness between the child and the parent often antedates the clinical presentation. The symptoms are grouped into physical complaints, irrational fears about the well-being of the parent, and fears concerning the child's own well-being.

Elliot presents with various **tics**. He demonstrates motor tics in the form of facial grimacing and eye blinking, and vocal tics in the form of grunting and barking. Tics are movements or noises, the production of which is outside of the person's control. Even though they are involuntary, the person is able, with concentration, to suppress them at times. Anxiety worsens the frequency and intensity of tics, while sleep and rest may cause their temporary disappearance. The progressive course of Elliot's symptoms is quite consistent with the diagnosis of **Tourette's disorder**. These tics may progress to involuntary shouting and utterance of obscenities, or they may remain static. High-potency neuroleptics, especially **pimozide**, provide some degree of relief. Tourette's disorder may be comorbid with ADHD. Administration of psychostimulants as treatment for ADHD may unmask a dormant tic disorder.

Items 168-176

Choose the **BEST** response.

168. All of the following statements are **TRUE** regarding ADHD **EXCEPT**:

    (A)   The disorder is fairly common, affecting about 5% of preschoolers.
    (B)   Girls are more likely to be affected than boys.
    (C)   The most common time for the diagnosis is elementary school.
    (D)   Conversion disorder, alcoholism, and antisocial personality disorder are common in families of children affected by ADHD.
    (E)   The symptoms first appear before age three.

169. Which of the following are **COMMON** clinical findings in children with ADHD?

    (A)   failure to pay attention to details, numerous careless mistakes
    (B)   failure to complete assignments
    (C)   inability to wait one's turn
    (D)   restlessness, fidgeting
    (E)   All of the above

170. All of the following are **TRUE** regarding etiologic and predisposing factors in ADHD **EXCEPT**:

    (A)   Genetic factors are implicated.
    (B)   Nonfocal neurologic findings may appear suggesting subtle brain damage.
    (C)   Additives, food colorings, and sugar may be responsible for the hyperactivity.
    (D)   Psychological factors, such as prolonged emotional deprivation, may be responsible for ADHD-like behaviors.
    (E)   Temperament may be a predisposing factor.

171. Clinical and laboratory findings **COMMONLY** found in children with ADHD include

    (A)   spike-and-wave pattern over the temporal lobe on the EEG
    (B)   abnormal continuous performance test
    (C)   abnormal lateral ventricles on CT scan
    (D)   A and C only
    (E)   A, B, and C

172. The treatment strategies for ADHD include all of the following **EXCEPT**:

   (A)   pharmacotherapy
   (B)   behavior modification techniques
   (C)   parent training sessions
   (D)   restriction of dietary sugar
   (E)   psychotherapy

173. All of the following drugs have been used for treatment of ADHD **EXCEPT**:

   (A)   pemoline
   (B)   methylphenidate
   (C)   pimozide
   (D)   dextroamphetamine
   (E)   clonidine

174. **COMMON** side effects associated with the use of methylphenidate include

   (A)   growth suppression
   (B)   insomnia
   (C)   nausea
   (D)   A and C only
   (E)   A, B, and C

175. Which of the following constitute a **RELATIVE** contraindication to the use of psychostimulants in the treatment of ADHD?

   (A)   comorbid depression and anxiety disorders
   (B)   presence of a tic disorder
   (C)   presence of other learning disabilities
   (D)   comorbid conduct disorder
   (E)   no contraindications exist for the use of psychostimulants

176. Which of the following classes of drugs used in the treatment of ADHD have been associated with several reports of sudden death in children?

   (A)   psychostimulants
   (B)   tricyclic antidepressants
   (C) α_1-agonists
   (D)   A and C only
   (E)   None of the above

ANSWERS AND TUTORIAL ON ITEMS 168-176

The answers are: **168-B; 169-E; 170-C; 171-B; 172-D; 173-C; 174-E; 175-B; 176-B**. **Attention-deficit/hyperactivity disorder** (ADHD) is fairly common. It is characterized by impairment in attention and concentration that are inconsistent with the child's age. Impulsivity and hyperactivity are the other characteristics of this syndrome. The reported incidence of ADHD is about **5%** of all preschool children, with a **male:female ratio of 5:1**. Although frequently evident prior to age three, ADHD is most commonly diagnosed in elementary school, when the social demand for sustained attention and concentration becomes important for academic performance. ADHD frequently coexists with other conditions, such as **learning disabilities** and **conduct disorder**. **Depression** and **anxiety disorders** also occur with ADHD.

In **families of children with ADHD**, one finds a greater incidence of attentional disorders, histories of conversion disorder in women, and alcoholism and sociopathy in men. The **etiology of ADHD** is unknown. There is some evidence of familial transmission. Monozygotic twins are more frequently affected than dizygotic twins. Parents of children with ADHD are more likely to have had the disorder themselves. The frequent presence of **nonfocal (soft) neurological findings** points to the possibility of subtle brain damage. While an EEG may show transient abnormalities, these are inconsistent and nonspecific. No structural abnormalities are detected by CT scans. By far, the most consistent abnormality found in children with ADHD is errors of omission on continuous performance testing.

Temperament, history of perinatal trauma, and history of prolonged emotional deprivation are among the **predisposing factors** to the development of ADHD. The later may manifest itself by hyperactivity, but the behavior tends to normalize when deprivation is relieved. Contrary to popular belief, food additives and sugar are neither associated with nor do they exacerbate ADHD.

The **treatment of ADHD** is multimodal. It requires both medications and psychotherapy. Careful coordination between the parents, doctors, and school is of paramount importance if the treatment is to be successful. Psychostimulants are the mainstay of pharmacotherapy. **Dextroamphetamine**, **methylphenidate**, and, less commonly, **pemoline** are considered first-line drugs in treatment of ADHD. All except pemoline are characterized by short half-life and are given twice daily, usually before and during school hours. The goal of pharmacotherapy is to improve school performance. The drugs are not given in the evening, on weekends, and holidays in order to minimize their side effects. Although these compounds are relatively safe, their use is associated with nausea, appetite suppression, insomnia, rebound hyperactivity, and transient growth suppression. Thus, drug holidays are important to assure the treated youngster reaches normal weight and height. Additionally, psychostimulants are known to bring on **tic disorders** in predisposed children and to exacerbate existing tic disorders. In cases of personal or family history of tic disorders, **clonidine**, an α_1-agonist, is the preferred drug. Similarly, psychosis may be exacerbated by the administration of amphetamine-like compounds.

Tricyclic antidepressants are second-line drugs in the treatment of ADHD. They are particularly effective in cases with comorbid anxiety or depressive disorders. The controversy surrounding the use of tricyclic antidepressants stems from several reports of sudden death. While the cause of death was not clearly determined, the possibility of tricyclic-induced arrhythmia was entertained. Special caution must be taken in prescribing these agents to children, with pretreatment EKGs and careful drug level monitoring required. **Pimozide** is a high-potency neuroleptic, used primarily in the treatment of **Tourette's disorder**. It plays no role in the management of ADHD.

Individual psychotherapy, behavior management, and parent training are important constituents of the overall **care of ADHD-affected children**. The focus of **individual psychotherapy** should be restoration and maintenance of self-esteem, so frequently lacking in a child whose academic and social performance is impaired. It can also assist in developing new social skills and improvement of impulse control. **Behavioral management** provides techniques for direct reinforcement of socially desirable behavior, and, thus, is helpful in managing the social sequelae of ADHD. Finally, **parent training** and family therapy assist the parents in handling difficult behaviors in a way that is neither punitive nor damaging, as well as addressing the parental difficulties of living with a hyperactive child.

CHAPTER V
DELIRIUM, DEMENTIA, AND PSYCHIATRIC MANIFESTATIONS OF AIDS

Items 177-182

Choose the **BEST** response.

177. All the following typically occur in delirium **EXCEPT**:

   (A)   fluctuating level of consciousness
   (B)   perceptual distortions, hallucinations
   (C)   sustained euphoria
   (D)   diminished attention/concentration
   (E)   disruptions of the sleep-wake cycle

178. Delirium

   (A)   occurs in 10-15% of all hospitalized medical/surgical patients
   (B)   is associated with a 40-50% one year mortality rate
   (C)   is especially common in postsurgical, elderly and ICU patients
   (D)   A and C only
   (E)   A, B, and C

179. The following abnormal physical findings may be associated with delirium

   (A)   elevated vital signs, including temperature
   (B)   frontal release signs (palmomental, Babinski, rooting reflexes)
   (C)   papilledema
   (D)   All of the above
   (E)   None of the above

180. Which of the following objective tests is abnormal during delirium from any cause

   (A)   CT of the head
   (B)   EEG (Electroencephalogram)
   (C)   Lumbar puncture
   (D)   EKG
   (E)   serum glucose

181. Frequent or common causes of delirium include all the following **EXCEPT**:

   (A) sepsis
   (B) focal lesions of the CNS (e.g., tumors)
   (C) electrolyte imbalances, especially low cations (Ca^{2+}, Mg^{2+})
   (D) drug intoxication or withdrawal
   (E) hypoxia

182. While treatment involves reversing the cause of the delirium, management of the delirious patient may also include

   (A) regulation of environmental stimulation (light and noise)
   (B) low doses of high potency antipsychotics
   (C) calming human contact with frequent orientation
   (D) A and C only
   (E) A, B, and C

ANSWERS AND TUTORIAL ON ITEMS 177-182

The answers are: **177-C; 178-E; 179-D; 180-B; 181-B; 182-E.** The syndrome of **delirium** occurs when global brain function is impaired from any cause. With a few rare exceptions, the impairment is acute and potentially reversible. The condition is often a medical emergency. Acute brain failure is as ominous as acute heart failure and requires similarly aggressive treatment.

The cardinal features of delirium are acute or subacute onset, fluctuations between alertness and drowsiness, disorientation, perceptual distortions and hallucinations, decreased attention/concentration, and incoherence. Motor restlessness and sleep-wake cycle disruption are also common, with patients sleeping in the daytime and up all night, or napping and waking throughout the twenty four hours. Agitation or paranoia frequently occur. Delirium may produce euphoria or any extreme mood, though anxiety is more typical. Prolonged mood elevation, however, is not common. Mood, like other symptoms, fluctuates, so that delirious patients move from one mood state to another, just as their consciousness shifts from alertness to sleep.

The 40-50% one year mortality associated with delirium, the link to hospitalization for severe illness (ICU), and the preponderance of elderly patients all underline the severity of this condition. Because the symptoms of delirium are psychiatric, and the condition is associated with stigmatized patients (elderly, mildly demented patients and alcoholics), medical personnel often fail to make the diagnosis. Delirium is an urgent medical situation that requires urgent attention.

Evaluation begins with a physical examination, including vital signs and fundoscopy. Elevated pulse, blood pressure and temperature are all common (especially in delirium secondary to infection or to sedative withdrawal). Frontal release signs, which may normalize with effective treatment, may be found. **Papilledema** is rare, but when present indicates increased intracranial pressure as the cause of the abnormal mental status. The **EEG** shows diffuse slowing in delirium from any cause. A more specific pattern (K complexes) occurs in delirium due to hepatic encephalopathy. All the other tests on the list are sometimes part of an evaluation for delirium, but relate to specific causes. The CT scan is probably the least useful, since delirium reflects metabolic more than structural pathology. An EKG will help diagnose delirium from severe arrhythmias leading to poor perfusion. Serum glucose is part of general metabolic screening and an lymphocyte profile is needed in any patient with AIDS or a possible CNS infection. It is not a routine part of the workup in the absence of other factors suggesting infection.

Focal CNS lesions, usually infarcts or tumors, do not typically present with delirium, which requires pervasive brain dysfunction. All the other conditions on the list--sepsis, cation deficiency, drug-related states and hypoxia--are high on the list of differential diagnosis of the causes of delirium.

Although reversing the underlying cause is the cornerstone of any treatment for delirium, mental status may not normalize immediately. Patients need to be managed carefully until they recover, to prevent self-injury. Manipulation of the environment by using light to encourage normal sleep-wake cycles and reducing meaningless background ("white") noise may help the patient be less confused. High potency antipsychotic drugs are best for reducing agitation and sedating patients, except those withdrawing from alcohol or sedatives. These patients need benzodiazepines or other cross-tolerant drugs to prevent delirium tremens (DTs). Finally, reassuring contact with familiar people can be of great help, particularly if the person knows to keep communication simple and concrete and is willing to repeat things over and over to help the delirious person stay oriented.

Items 183-187

Choose the **BEST** response.

183. The diagnosis of dementia

  (A)   Requires either disorientation or at least three other intellectual deficits (impairment of language, problem solving, judgment, orientation, attention/concentration).
  (B)   Excludes the diagnosis of delirium in the same patient.
  (C)   Requires evidence of decline from a previous baseline, with impairment of social or occupational functioning.
  (D)   A and C only
  (E)   A, B, and C

184. The "Four As" of dementia, one of which must be present for diagnosis, include all of the following **EXCEPT**:

  (A)   anxiety
  (B)   apraxia
  (C)   agnosia
  (D)   aphasia
  (E)   abstraction (diminished)

185. In dementia

  (A)   general personality function is well-preserved
  (B)   hallucinations and delusions are quite rare
  (C)   sleep-wake cycles are often disrupted
  (D)   A and C only
  (E)   A, B, and C

186. DSM-IV further requires that the cause of the dementia be specified, when known. Rank the causes of dementia, from **MOST to LEAST** common

  (A)   vascular insufficiency, Alzheimer's disease, HIV or related infection, head injury, Vitamin B_{12} deficiency
  (B)   HIV or related infection, vascular insufficiency, head injury, Alzheimer's disease, Vitamin B_{12} deficiency
  (C)   Alzheimer's disease, vascular insufficiency, head injury, HIV or related infection, Vitamin B_{12} deficiency
  (D)   vascular disease, HIV or related infection, Vitamin B_{12} deficiency, Alzheimer's disease, head injury
  (E)   head injury, Alzheimer's disease, vascular disease, HIV or related infection, Vitamin B_{12} deficiency

187. The **MOST** common form of dementia

  (A)   accounts for 50-60% of all cases of dementia
  (B)   occurs in about 30% of people who reach age sixty
  (C)   occurs in about 65% of people who reach age 85
  (D)   A and C only
  (E)   A, B, and C

ANSWERS AND TUTORIAL ON ITEMS 183-187

The answers are: **183-C; 184-A; 185-C; 186-C; 187-A**. **Dementia** is a clinical syndrome of persistent (though occasionally reversible) multiple cognitive and functional deficits related to known or suspected brain pathology. The diagnosis requires **memory impairment** and **one** of aphasia, apraxia, agnosia, or disturbance of executive functioning (planning, sequencing, abstraction). The person must also have deteriorated from a previous level of social or occupational functioning. Delirium may be superimposed on dementia; indeed, demented patients readily become delirious when ill. The diagnostic criteria require only that the deficits of demented patients do not occur exclusively in the course of a delirium.

Although dementia is defined by the **loss of cognitive abilities**, changes in personality, affective dysregulation and psychotic symptoms all may occur. Hallucinations occur in 20-30% of Alzheimer's disease patients and delusions (usually persecutory) in 30-40%. Extreme or disinhibited mood states are present in 40-50% of this group, with 10-20% having a full blown depressive disorder. Sleep-wake cycle changes--fragmented sleep and nocturnal worsening (sundowning)--are also characteristic.

Clinicians using DSM-IV must specify the cause of the dementia whenever possible. Although particular clinical features help differentiate one from another (see below), verifying the etiology of a dementia may require knowledge of tissue pathology not available in life. Epidemiological information about the relative frequency of and risk factors for different dementias is therefore essential for identifying the cause of dementia in patients who present for initial evaluation.

Alzheimer's disease accounts for 50-60% of all cases of dementia. It afflicts roughly 5% of the general population who reach age 65 and 15-25% of those 85 or older. Vascular dementia, the next most common form, accounts for 15-30% of dementias; 10-15% of demented patients have both problems. (DSM-IV allows the diagnosis of dementia from multiple or mixed causes. The residual category of dementia not otherwise specified applies only when the cause(s) cannot be identified.)

Head trauma, normal pressure hydrocephalus, alcohol-related brain damage (including thiamine deficiency) and mass lesions (tumor, abscess, hematoma) account for 1-5% of all dementias. Movement disorders (Huntington's disease, Parkinson's disease), AIDS and collagen vascular diseases with vasculitis cause about 1%. Causes such as Creutzfeldt-Jakob disease, viral encephalitis, Vitamin B_{12} or folate deficiency, endocrine disease, inborn errors of metabolism (e.g., Wilson's disease), neurosyphilis, meningitis, or severe renal insufficiency are rare (less than 1%) but worth identifying because some are potentially reversible.

Items 188-198

Choose the **BEST** response.

188. All the following implicate decreased acetylcholine activity as a cause of Alzheimer's disease **EXCEPT**:

   (A)   degeneration of the nucleus basalis of Meynert
   (B)   decreased concentration of acetylcholine and choline acetyltransferase in brain tissue
   (C)   decrease in locus ceruleus neurons
   (D)   transient improvement with physostigmine and arecoline
   (E)   transient worsening with scopolamine or atropine

189. Other abnormalities under investigation in Alzheimer's disease include:

   (A)   overproduction of β/A4 amyloid precursor protein
   (B)   increased frequency of presence of the apolipoprotein E4 gene
   (C)   rigidity of neuronal cell membranes, possibly due to abnormal phospholipid metabolism
   (D)   A and C
   (E)   A, B, and C

Items 190-194

Matching

Profound, late stage dementias all look roughly the same. Earlier in the illness, however, certain symptoms or objective findings can differentiate one form from another. Match the causes of dementia in the items below with the unique, **MOST** differentiating clinical features in the answers.

   (A)   Insidious onset, continuous, gradual progression; patient often unconcerned or unaware of deficits; shallow, labile affect; widened sulci and enlarged ventricles on neuroimaging studies.

   (B)   Incontinence and shuffling gait when cognitive impairment is still relatively mild; history of subarachnoid hemorrhage.

   (C)   Stepwise progression; focal neurologic and frontal release signs early in the course; white matter lesions on MRI scan.

(D)   Marked tics or choreoathetoid movements when language, memory, and insight are only mildly to moderately impaired; prominence of psychotic or depressive symptoms; deterioration of the caudate nucleus on CT scan ("butterfly pattern").

(E)   Bradykinesia, cogwheel rigidity, abnormal gait; markedly slow thinking; apathy, depression.

(F)   Acute or subacute onset; marked sadness or apathy; cognitive deficits found on mental status examination less severe than those reported by the patient; variable performance on tasks of similar difficulty; early loss of social skills; patients emphasize their failures and disability, make little effort to perform simple tasks.

190.   Dementia due to Parkinson's disease

191.   Vascular dementia

192.   Dementia of the Alzheimer's type

193.   Dementia due to normal pressure hydrocephalus

194.   Dementia due to Huntington's disease

Choose the **BEST** response.

195.   Potentially reversible causes of dementia include:

(A)   normal pressure hydrocephalus
(B)   major depressive episode
(C)   thiamine or other vitamin deficiency
(D)   All of the above
(E)   None of the above

196.   If a patient's clinical presentation or mental status examination suggests dementia, subsequent work-up includes all the following **EXCEPT**:

(A)   EEG
(B)   imaging study, preferably MRI
(C)   serum chemistries, screen for collagen vascular disease, CBC
(D)   HIV, VDRL or RPR, possible lumbar puncture
(E)   measurement of thyroid function, Vitamin B_{12} and folate levels

197. Neuropsychological testing may be useful

  (A)   to document the patient's functional baseline, so changes can be followed more precisely
  (B)   to differentiate "subcortical" from "cortical" or depressive patterns of cognitive impairment
  (C)   to evaluate subtle impairment of competence for legal purposes
  (D)   A and C only
  (E)   A, B, and C

198. Treatment of established dementia from any cause is symptomatic and supportive. Typical interventions include all the following **EXCEPT**:

  (A)   Developing simple routines for patients that involve frequent orientation, regular toileting, consistent meal and bedtimes, regular social contact.
  (B)   Education of caretakers and family members.
  (C)   Regular support groups for family members and caretakers, sometimes including family therapy to reduce conflict among multiple caretakers and encourage ongoing involvement by multiple family members.
  (D)   High dose, high potency antipsychotic drugs to control agitation and prevent violence.
  (E)   Antidepressant and antianxiety drugs in low or regular clinical dosages for affective symptoms when present.

ANSWERS AND TUTORIAL ON ITEMS 188-198

The answers are: **188-C; 189-E; 190-E; 191-C; 192-A; 193-B; 194-D; 195-D; 196-A; 197-E; 198-D**. The puzzle of **Alzheimer's disease** has received the lion's share of research attention in the field of dementia. Current theory implicates a diffuse loss of acetylcholine (ACH) activity throughout the cortex, possibly secondary to degeneration of the nucleus basalis of Meynert, where ACH-containing cell bodies cluster. These cells have especially rich projections to the hippocampus, consistent with the prominence of memory impairment in Alzheimer's disease. The irregular, patchy distribution of the cortical lesions accounts for the variable onset of particular symptoms in different patients. That is, location of the secondary cortical lesions may explain why some patients have prominent language problems early on, others lose judgment, and still others develop paranoid delusions. As the lesions become more widespread, all patients have multiple deficits.

Low levels of brain ACH and its synthetic enzymes are consistent with this model, as are the transient positive effects of cholinergic drugs (physostigmine and arecoline) and the negative impact of anticholinergic agents (atropine, scopolamine). The loss of locus ceruleus neurons seen in Alzheimer's disease points to other possible contributory mechanisms, specifically decreased noradrenergic function. The association of Alzheimer's disease with overproduction of β/A4 amyloid precursor protein, the presence of an apolipoprotein E4 gene, and with abnormal membrane function all suggest that decreased ACH activity does not account for all the pathological changes and clinical features of the disease. Further basic research will likely elucidate the genetic pathology underlying this often hereditary condition.

Although the final diagnosis of the cause of dementia requires tissue examination, certain clinical features differentiate some causes from others. Like Alzheimer's disease, the dementia associated with Huntington's disease and Parkinson's disease may represent cortical dysfunction secondary to loss of subcortical input. In Huntington's disease, the caudate nucleus degenerates, producing choreoathetoid movements and tics. Parkinson's disease, characterized by loss of dopaminergic cells in the substantia nigra, also presents with early motor signs (bradykinesia, rigidity, cogwheeling, shuffling gait). Dementia, a late complication in 20 to 30% of people with Parkinson's disease, is often characterized by slowed thought, analogous to the slowed motor behavior. Before the role of the nucleus basalis of Meynert was fully appreciated, Parkinson's and Huntington's diseases were called "subcortical" dementias, highlighting the relative prominence of motor signs, the early mood and personality changes, the relative preservation of certain cognitive abilities (i.e., calculation, recognition, use of language despite dysarthria), and related neuropsychological test findings. As noted above, it now appears that Alzheimer's disease originates in subcortical cell bodies. Still, the clinical distinction between subcortical and cortical dementia remains valid, although the terminology is somewhat misleading.

In the matching items, answer B presents the classical triad of normal pressure hydrocephalus: shuffling gait, incontinence and dementia. Depression and akinesis, even mutism, may occur. This condition results from blockage of the normal drainage of CSF, usually a late sequela of subarachnoid hemorrhage. On CT or MRI scan, the patient will have enlarged ventricles with compressed but not atrophied cortex. CSF pressure, measured via lumbar puncture, is normal. Shunting to relieve the pressure in the ventricles may dramatically restore function, if done within a year or so of onset of the problem. Later, the condition becomes irreversible.

Alzheimer's disease by definition has an insidious onset with gradual, continuous progression. Cognitive and language dysfunction occur early, with motor dysfunction and cortical release signs only appearing after diffuse cortical damage has occurred. Affective symptoms, though possible, are not prominent--patients often seem unaware of their deficits and inappropriately cheerful, especially in the middle stage of the disease. On mental status they often confabulate, give haphazard answers, and are pleased with any preserved ability. This contrasts with the mental status findings in patients with cognitive loss secondary to depression (description F). These patients often have a prior history of depression or bipolar disorder. They are dysphoric and deeply concerned about any possible impairment, even though they perform relatively well on mental status examination. They will give frequent "don't know" or "I can't" answers, and zero in on every failure. The syndrome is partially reversible with antidepressants or electoconvulsive therapy (ECT)--mild, residual cognitive deficits are common but the patients may be able to function normally once the depressive features remit.

Vascular dementia occurs in stepwise fashion, with occlusive events leading to sudden new losses of function. A history of heart disease, arrhythmias, diabetes, or hypertension is common. Patients develop frontal release and localizing neurologic signs relatively early. The deficits observed will correlate with the location of the lesions seen on MRI (but often not CT) scans. Although the changes of vascular dementia are irreversible, early recognition and aggressive treatment for cardiovascular disease may slow progression of the illness.

It is important to remember that non-Alzheimer's dementias may stabilize or improve with specific treatment. Advanced dementia from any cause is irreversible, but early recognition and treatment of depression, vitamin deficiency, normal pressure hydrocephalus, metabolic, endocrine or collagen vascular disorders, uncontrolled hypertension, and renal disease can preserve patients' functional capacity and independence. Thus, the work-up for dementia requires searching for rare but treatable causes. A comprehensive work-up involves physical and mental status examination, an imaging study, and measurement of usual chemistries, plus thyroid function tests, screens for HIV, syphilis, collagen vascular disease, and vitamin deficiency. In contrast to delirium, an EEG is not generally useful--EEG changes in dementia usually don't occur until the later, irreversible stages. A complete work-up need be done only once, although patients with previously diagnosed irreversible dementia can acquire a second exacerbating condition such as drug toxicity, nutritional deficiency, or infection. Additional insults or secondary delirium should be suspected and treated if the Alzheimer's patient suddenly worsens or demonstrates atypical progression of symptoms.

Neuropsychological testing can be indicated in dementia for all the reasons given. With many clinicians typically treating a patient over the course of a dementing disease, an objectively determined baseline can help identify atypical features early, allowing for appropriate and sometimes ameliorating treatments. Facing the likelihood of relentless progression also requires early attention to the issues of competence and advance directives. Patients need to order their affairs while they still can and make their wishes about treatment clear. Psychological testing can help ensure these decisions will be honored when patients can no longer state them and also prevent the implementation of inappropriate decisions made by incompetent patients.

Because so little can be done to arrest the progression of disease in the dementing patient, the clinician should attend to the environmental and social factors that determine how long the patient may be able to live independently or in a sheltered setting short of a nursing home. Making the environment simple, safe, routine, and pleasantly stimulating can forestall many of the complications that wear out caretakers and lead to institutionalization. Incontinence, sleeplessness, agitation and disorganized behavior, rather than cognitive impairment, are what make demented people so hard to live with. Many can improve with attention to the immediate environment and correction of sensory deficits (glasses or cataract surgery for impaired vision; hearing aids for deafness).

The care of a demented person burdens family members severely. Education can reduce dangerous misunderstandings, for example that the person is willfully acting withdrawn or socially inappropriate, or that the patient must be tied up to prevent wandering away. Support groups run by hospitals or the Alzheimer's Disease Association help families mourn, share the heavy burdens of care, and learn about appropriate resources such as respite care (temporary, elective nursing home placement). Support groups may prevent what is often a single family member from becoming unduly isolated by the demands of caregiving, and succumbing to illness or depression because of it.

The best way to prevent caregiver burnout is to create a network of multiple caregivers-- this may require counselling or therapy for an individual family, both to underline the recommendation that this occur and to reduce conflicts that typically result. Medications that help with management include antidepressants (especially those without anticholinergic side-effects) and, occasionally, antianxiety agents for relevant symptoms. (Patients often do not tolerate the sedative effects of antianxiety drugs very well). Methylphenidate, while not commonly used for depression in other populations, may be particularly helpful for those with mild dementia, improving alertness and mood without anticholinergic side-effects. High potency antipsychotic drugs are also often used, but only in very low doses (roughly one tenth the dose given to patients with schizophrenia). They can reduce agitation, moderate hallucinations and delusions when present, and safely sedate patients at night.

94

Patient I. A 65-year-old woman with a high school education is brought in by her family because of six months of deteriorating social functioning and memory loss. The patient is in good health except for maturity-onset diabetes mellitus, diagnosed a year ago. She uses oral hypoglycemic agents and admits to frequent dietary lapses. The patient retired from an office job around the time her problems started. She has lost roughly 15 pounds, and she can sleep only 3 or 4 hours, most nights. She is most impaired in the morning, agitated, wringing her hands, and saying she knows she belongs in a nursing home but would rather die than go there. Her speech is slow and monotonous but syntactically correct. On mental status examination she is alert and oriented, can recall only one object at three minutes spontaneously but remembers two more with prompting, and refuses serial calculations and digit span. She can spell world forward and backward and follow two step directions. Abstraction is partly diminished. Long-term memory is basically intact.

199. The **MOST** likely diagnosis is

   (A) dementia of the Alzheimer's type
   (B) vascular dementia
   (C) pseudodementia
   (D) benign senescent forgetfulness
   (E) delirium from unregulated diabetes mellitus

200. Intervention should include

   (A) CBC, serum chemistries including measurement of thyroid function, glycosylated hemoglobin, and a glucose tolerance test
   (B) EEG
   (C) initiation of treatment with an antidepressant
   (D) A and C only
   (E) A, B, and C

Patient II. At his annual physical examination, a 75-year-old man expresses concern over the gradual decline in his memory in the past few years. He has to write down phone numbers and lists of things he formerly remembered easily, and it takes him a long time to recall people's names. His mood is generally good, he sleeps well most nights, and he can still enjoy reading, attending plays and movies, and gardening. The physician notes that the patient was able to get dressed easily after being examined. He is normotensive with no pathological reflexes or focal neurologic findings. He is oriented to person, place and time, recalls 3/4 objects at five minutes, can perform serial calculations slowly but accurately, and has no problem naming objects or repeating sentences. He can abstract categories and interpret proverbs. Remote memory is intact, but he has to consult a notebook to give the names and dosages of his medications.

201. The **MOST** likely diagnosis is

   (A) dementia of the Alzheimer's type
   (B) pseudodementia
   (C) malingering
   (D) benign senescent forgetfulness
   (E) vascular dementia

202. Intervention should include

   (A) serum chemistries, CBC, vitamin levels and thyroid function tests
   (B) methylphenidate
   (C) counsel that his condition will likely progress and give advice to begin to order his affairs and consider writing an advance directive
   (D) A and C only
   (E) A, B, and C

Patient III. A homosexual man describes his 32-year-old, college educated partner of having had a personality change over the previous six months. The man has become moody, withdrawn, and slovenly. He sleeps more than he used to and seems to have little appetite. Lately, he has become suspicious, accusing his lover of infidelity for no reason. Physical examination, including normal gait, is remarkable only for signs of oral thrush. On mental status examination, the patient is alert, but guarded and with slowed psychomotor function. He is oriented to place and year but misses the date by two days. He can recall only 1 of 3 objects at five minutes, even with prompting. He remembers 4 digits forward and two in reverse. He can name the past three presidents only. He has difficulty following a two step command and cannot name the parts of a watch.

203. The **MOST** likely diagnosis is

   (A) schizotypal personality disorder
   (B) AIDS-related dementia
   (C) delirium secondary to viral encephalitis
   (D) Alzheimer's dementia with presenile onset
   (E) dementia from normal pressure hydrocephalus

204. Intervention should include

   (A) serum chemistries, including CBC, HIV test, RPR and hepatitis screen
   (B) lumbar puncture
   (C) neuroimaging study
   (D) A and C only
   (E) A, B, and C

Patient IV. A 35-year-old woman with Down's syndrome (trisomy 21) is brought in by her family. She had previously learned to read street signs and write her name. Until a year ago, she attended a sheltered workshop where she sorted color coded components for appliance repair. In the past year, she has become more impaired and can no longer reliably recognize people she does not see every day. She cannot dress herself as she used to. She is unable to work. On mental status examination, she is pleasant but distracted and oriented to person only. Her speech is grammatically fragmented and dysarthric. She cannot remember what she ate for lunch an hour before. She does not recognize a picture of a stop sign.

205.   The **MOST** likely diagnosis is

(A)   mental retardation secondary to Down's syndrome
(B)   dementia of the Alzheimer's type
(C)   oppositional defiant disorder
(D)   dependent personality disorder
(E)   pseudodementia

ANSWERS AND TUTORIAL ON ITEMS 199-205

The answers are: **199-C; 200-D; 201-D; 202-A; 203-B; 204-E; 205-B**. **Patient I** is a typical case of pseudodementia or depression-related cognitive impairment. The patient has a subacute onset following an identifiable life event; her mood and vegetative functioning are consistent with depression. Her diurnal mood variation helps differentiate depression and dementia-- demented patients worsen in the latter part of the day; depressed patients are often worse in the early morning hours. This patient complains of problems more severe than those revealed on mental status examination; she gives "I can't" responses, and she has no language disorder. No apraxia or agnosia are mentioned. Noninsulin-dependent diabetes mellitus is not typically associated with either severe hypoglycemia or ketoacidosis. The patient is at risk for accelerated cardiovascular disease, but not within the first year of diagnosis of her diabetes. She has more complaints and functional impairment than implied by the diagnosis of benign senescent forgetfulness. This patient, like any other with altered mental status, should undergo a basic screening evaluation, with special attention to maximizing treatment for any current medical problems. She does not need an EEG, as she is not delirious. Treatment with an antidepressant would have a high probability of restoring her to her previous level of functioning, though mild cognitive deficits may remain even if she responds well.

    Patient II is exhibiting **benign senescent forgetfulness**. Some decrease in short-term memory and recall is a normal part of aging. The problem is not a disorder and has no place in DSM-IV. The patient is not aphasic (can name and repeat) or apraxic (dresses easily). Agnosia is not described. He has no reported illness associated with dementia, including no hypertension predictive of vascular dementia. His mental status is fine, except for the short-term memory deficit, and he is not functionally impaired. His ability to abstract and to compensate using lists indicates that his problem solving (executive) abilities are intact. Because of his age, he could be in the early stages of a more serious dementing process, so inexpensive screening is indicated. However, the most important intervention is reassurance that his condition is not necessarily a progressive dementia. He does not require any treatment.

Patient III probably has AIDS dementia. Although personality change is the presenting complaint, evaluation reveals the classic deficits of dementia [short-term memory impairment, decreased attention/concentration, decreased language capacity (aphasia) and decreased executive functioning (not able to follow complex commands)]. His poor self-care, suspiciousness, and sleep disorder, while not diagnostic of dementia, are consistent with it. Schizotypal personality disorder does not begin in middle age. His normal gait is evidence against normal pressure hydrocephalus. Delirium is a possibility, though the history of six months of gradual decline and the lack of physical findings make it less likely than dementia, especially since the patient does not exhibit fluctuating level of consciousness. Alzheimer's disease can begin prior to age 65, a condition once called "presenile dementia." However, the patient has a major risk factor for AIDS (homosexuality) and a classic manifestation (oral thrush). The initial presentation of AIDS is often a psychiatric disorder.

Evaluation of mental status changes in a patient with possible AIDS includes specialized serum studies, neuroimaging and a lumbar puncture. The latter will allow for diagnosis of specific opportunistic, sometimes treatable infections of the nervous system. HIV itself can infect the nervous system and cause a dementia which, if discovered early, may be partially reversible with antiviral therapy.

Patient IV is an example of a person with trisomy 21 who has survived into middle age, and, as is almost universal for such patients, has now developed **Alzheimer's disease**. Although this patient was suffering from mental retardation at baseline, she now warrants a diagnosis of dementia because her functional level has markedly decreased. She has classic symptoms including decreased language capacity, agnosia, apraxia, and loss of short-term memory. She is not depressed, ruling out pseudodementia. Oppositional defiant disorder and dependent personality disorder do not begin in adulthood. In any case, she is not oppositional, just incapacitated.

Items 206-209

Choose the **BEST** response.

206. Which of the following is **NOT** a method of transmission of HIV?

    (A)   intravenous drug abuse
    (B)   mother-infant transplacental transmission
    (C)   unprotected homosexual intercourse
    (D)   unprotected heterosexual intercourse
    (E)   masturbation

207. Which of the following is **TRUE** about HIV infection?

   (A)   The most common sign of early infection is clinical depression.
   (B)   CNS infection is virtually universal and occurs early in the course of the disease.
   (C)   The acute phase of infection lasts on average nine years.
   (D)   CD8 T-lymphocytes are the usual target.
   (E)   The latency stage of infection lasts up to six months.

208. The diagnosis of AIDS in an HIV positive person is made when

   (A)   The patient develops *Pneumocystis carinii* pneumonia.
   (B)   CD4 T-lymphocyte count is less than 500 cells/mm^3.
   (C)   The patient develops *Toxoplasma gondii* infection.
   (D)   A and C only.
   (E)   A, B, and C

209. All of the following are neuropsychiatric aspects of HIV-related brain disease **EXCEPT**:

   (A)   body dysmorphic disorder
   (B)   cognitive impairment
   (C)   bipolar disorder
   (D)   delirium
   (E)   psychosis

ANSWERS AND TUTORIAL ON ITEMS 206-209

The answers are: **206-E; 207-B; 208-D; 209-A**. The **human immunodeficiency virus (HIV) infection** that was first detected in the early 1980's and has reached epidemic proportions, is transmitted through **exchange of body fluids,** such as blood and semen. Although isolated in vaginal secretions and saliva, HIV is not particularly infective in that exchange. The largest group currently infected are homosexual men, followed by intravenous drug abusers. HIV can also be transmitted in heterosexual intercourse, the predominant mode of transmission in Africa. It is also a growing mode in the US. Other groups at risk for transmission are infants born to infected mothers, hemophiliacs who have received blood products prior to the institution of rigorous testing, and patients who have received contaminated blood. The sexual behaviors that pose the greatest risks are unprotected anal, oral and vaginal intercourse. Kissing and masturbation are safe as long as there are no open sores.

   HIV infects a number of tissues in the body. Its primary target is the **CD4 T-lymphocyte.** The virus attaches to the cell membrane, gains entry into the cell, is transcribed by reverse transcriptase into DNA and becomes incorporated into human DNA. HIV is also neurotoxic, with CNS infection occurring early in the course of the disease. In fact, a number of patients report a period of cognitive slowing and confusion corresponding to the early acute stage of infection. The ability of HIV to cause severe subcortical dementia is well-known. The course of infection is divided into several stages. The first, called the initial or acute stage, spans the moment of infection to the development of antibodies. It can last from several weeks to months, but averages two months. During this stage, a patient might experience an acute meningoencephalitis or flu-like illness, followed by full recovery. The next phase is latency. It starts at the moment of seroconversion and lasts until development of the first opportunistic infection or other sign of AIDS, such as a CD4 count of less than 200 cells per cubic millimeter. This stage is asymptomatic and may last years, with the average being seven to nine years. The development of symptoms heralds the symptomatic phase that lasts until death.

Acquired immune deficiency syndrome (AIDS) is diagnosed in HIV-positive patients when **opportunistic infections** develop, such as *Pneumocystis carinii* or *Toxoplasma gondii*. Certain cancers, such as **Kaposi's sarcoma** and CNS lymphoma, also constitute grounds for the diagnosis of AIDS. Other criteria include HIV encephalopathy or a CD4 T-lymphocyte count less than 200 cells/mm3.

The **neuropsychiatric manifestations** of AIDS are numerous. They may include cognitive impairments that are transient and correspond to the acute phase of the illness. Additionally, delirium, either as a direct effect of the virus on the CNS, or as a result of other HIV-related CNS infections or treatments, is common. Subcortical dementia develops progressively throughout the course of the disease. There are cases of HIV brain disease that first manifest themselves by the acute onset of mania or psychosis. Body dysmorphic disorder is a near-delusional conviction that a minor defect or body part is grossly malformed and is hideously obvious. It is not common in HIV brain disease.

Items 210-214

Bob is a 35-year-old, HIV-positive, homosexual man who is referred for psychiatric evaluation by his internist, due to increase in confusion, forgetfulness and occasional complaints of clumsiness. Bob has begun to notice these changes over the past several months. While slow to develop, they do not seem to go away, and if anything, are getting worse. Bob is concerned about having to give up his job and has also noticed himself feeling depressed. Bob's lover wonders if this is a manifestation of AIDS.

Choose the **BEST** response.

210.   The psychiatrist, after conducting a psychiatric interview, should request

      (A)   a recent CD4 T-lymphocyte count
      (B)   the results of recent neuroimaging tests (MRI or CT)
      (C)   the results of recent neurologic examination
      (D)   A and C only
      (E)   A, B, and C

211. Having received the results of MRI of the head that show mild cerebral atrophy, but no evidence of masses, the psychiatrist turns to the neurologic examination. Which of the following neurological findings would support a presumptive diagnosis of early subcortical dementia?

    (A)   tremor
    (B)   decreased vibratory sense in lower extremities
    (C)   weakness in lower extremities
    (D)   A and C only
    (E)   A, B, and C

212. All of the following are consistent with the neuropsychological findings in early AIDS dementia complex **EXCEPT**:

    (A)   dense amnesia
    (B)   decreased concentration and attention
    (C)   visuospatial perceptual deficits
    (D)   dysarthria
    (E)   apathy

213. All of the following are consistent with the motor symptoms found in AIDS dementia complex **EXCEPT**:

    (A)   festinating gait
    (B)   bladder and bowel incontinence
    (C)   spastic weakness
    (D)   paraplegia
    (E)   hyperreflexia

214. Having made a diagnosis of AIDS dementia complex, the appropriate actions of the psychiatrist should include all of the following **EXCEPT**:

    (A)   Discuss it with Bob.
    (B)   Arrange for a joint meeting with Bob and his partner.
    (C)   Reassure Bob that the dementia is static and will not impair his ability to work.
    (D)   Assess the degree of functional impairment that Bob has.
    (E)   Evaluate the presence of depression and other reversible causes of cognitive decline.

ANSWERS AND TUTORIAL ON ITEMS 210-214

The answers are: **210-E; 211-D; 212-A; 213-A; 214-C**. Since HIV is a **neurotoxic virus** and the invasion of the CNS takes place early in the course of the infection, it is not surprising that neuropsychiatric manifestations may be the first sign of AIDS. The early symptoms of cognitive decline associated with HIV tend to be mild cognitive slowing, occasional confusion and forgetfulness. These symptoms progress to full-blown AIDS dementia complex in approximately 85% of patients. AIDS dementia is a subcortical dementia which manifests itself by motor, cognitive, and psychological symptoms. In the evaluation of dementia it is important to rule out other causes of cognitive decline, specifically CNS infections, tumors and hemorrhages. A recent CD4 T lymphocyte count is important in this assessment since cognitive symptoms are common in patients with counts less that 200 cells per cubic mm. Additionally, the workup should include CNS neuroimaging in search of abscesses, tumors, strokes and hemorrhages. Thorough physical and neurological examinations are important both in ruling out other conditions and in delineating neurologic findings that accompany subcortical dementias. A CT or MRI in patients with AIDS dementia typically shows mild, diffuse cortical atrophy which is nonspecific and, therefore, not diagnostic.

Early neurologic findings in AIDS dementia are nonspecific and reflect the diffuse nature of the pathologic process. Tremors, lower extremity weakness, clumsiness, dysarthria, forgetfulness, and impairments in attention and concentration are common. Noted also are visuospatial perceptual deficits. The memory loss involves short-term deficits rather than dense amnesia. However, intellectual functioning is well-preserved until late into the disease process. Sensory deficits, especially in the lower extremities, while quite common in AIDS patients due to HIV peripheral neuropathy, are not associated with dementia. As the dementia progresses, parapareses, quadriplegia, urinary and fecal incontinence are common. The muscular weakness tends to be spastic, with hyperreflexia and myoclonus. Seizures are seen late in the course of the illness. While ataxia is common, festinating gait is a specific finding associated with Parkinson's disease and not with AIDS dementia.

Personality changes are by far the most common first signs of early dementia. The patient may present with apathy, social withdrawal and emotional blunting. This presentation is frequently mistaken for depression. Later symptoms include inflexibility in thinking, erratic behavior, poor judgement, and abnormalities of speech. Suspiciousness, delusions, and hallucinations occur late in the disease process.

Management of the AIDS patient who presents with the early symptoms of cognitive deterioration requires a thorough medical, neurologic, and psychiatric assessment, including the above-mentioned tests. Neuropsychological testing helps establish a cognitive baseline. Honest discussion with the patient is of paramount importance. It is essential to establish a good working relationship with the patient, so as to be of help when the condition worsens. It is equally important to tell patients that while no specific treatments are available to preserve cognitive function, medications to improve mood and ameliorate psychotic symptoms are available. This counseling should include the patient's partner, who will likely be in a position to take care of the patient. Other issues of importance to address are the relatively slow decline of memory, intelligence and capacity to be productive. Hope is an important element to maintain. Finally, a durable power of attorney for decision-making should be discussed while the patient is still fully competent to designate the person who will act in his/her best interests, should incapacity strike.

215. A patient with known HIV seropositivity develops social withdrawal, sad mood, loss of sleep and appetite, poor concentration, and lack of interest in pleasurable activities. You diagnose a major depressive episode. The **MOST** appropriate treatment would be

    (A)   brief interpersonal psychotherapy
    (B)   fluoxetine
    (C)   nortriptyline
    (D)   A and C only
    (E)   A, B, and C

216. Which of the following neuroleptics is **MOST** useful in the management of psychosis in patients with AIDS?

    (A)   clozapine
    (B)   haloperidol
    (C)   chlorpromazine
    (D)   olanzapine
    (E)   trifluoperazine

217. Which of the following is **TRUE** regarding the use of benzodiazepines in patients with HIV brain disease?

    (A)   In view of the fact that AIDS is uniformly fatal, dependence on benzodiazepines is not of clinical significance.
    (B)   It is natural to feel anxious when afflicted with a terminal disease, therefore no pharmacological treatment of anxiety is necessary. It is more prudent to use psychotherapy for this purpose.
    (C)   Benzodiazepines must be administered in low dosages. Care should be taken to choose drugs with short half-life and few active metabolites.
    (D)   Diazepam, owing to its long half-life, is the drug of choice, since it prevents withdrawal symptoms upon discontinuation of use.
    (E)   Buspirone is as effective as benzodiazepines in the treatment of acute anxiety and is not addictive.

218. Which of the following is **TRUE** about the psychiatric aspects of AIDS?

    (A)   ECT is contraindicated in psychotically depressed AIDS patients.
    (B)   Hypochondriasis is common.
    (C)   Depression is not more common in AIDS patients than in the general papulation.
    (D)   Mania in AIDS patients my be related to the CNS infection itself or be related to the side-effects of antiviral agents.
    (E)   B and D only

The answers are: **215-D; 216-B; 217-C; 218-E. Depression** is common in patients with HIV regardless of their medical status. Moreover, untreated depression further worsens the functional impairment that AIDS patients may already experience. Treatment of depression should be multimodal and include psychotherapy and antidepressant medications. Brief interpersonal psychotherapy is especially appropriate for depression associated with loss. Pharmacotherapy in HIV brain disease must take into account that the impaired CNS is highly sensitive to medication and its side-effects. Thus, the rules applicable to geriatric psychopharmacology are true for patients with HIV brain disease. Anticholinergic medications should be avoided, as they increase the likelihood of delirium. Medication with a short half-life is preferable, since potential adverse effects will not linger as long as with long-acting medications. The doses of standard medications must be reduced and adjustments made slowly. Following these principles, nortriptyline has been the antidepressant of choice due to its low anticholinergic activity. Alternatively, short-acting **serotonin-specific reuptake inhibitors** (SSRIs) are being used frequently. Fluoxetine, with its very long half-life, is not a first choice drug. Methylphenidate also provides a good alternative or augmenting agent.

Among the **neuroleptics**, the principles of their use in AIDS patients remain the same as for any other patient. Agents with low anticholinergic activity, such as haloperidol, are preferred. It is important to remember that an average starting dose of haloperidol for the patient with AIDS must be 0.5-2.0 mg. AIDS patients are exquisitely sensitive to extrapyramidal side-effects. In the future, atypical antipsychotics with few extrapyramidal side-effects may supersede haloperidol, but research documenting their efficacy in AIDS is not yet available.

Benzodiazepines play an important role in management of anxiety spectrum disorders in the HIV-positive population. Dependence is an issue, just as it is with any patient, especially in light of the increasing life span of AIDS patients due to use of antiviral agents and protease inhibitors. Withdrawal is of concern with the discontinuation of any benzodiazepines, although the ones with long half-life tend to produce less florid symptomatology. The choice of benzodiazepine for an AIDS patient must include short half-life and absence of active metabolites. One needs to keep in mind the possible adverse effect on memory and cognitive function of benzodiazepines. Buspirone, while it may be useful in the management of generalized anxiety, is not particularly effective in panic attacks, or acute anxiety from any cause, because of its long response latency (delayed onset of action).

As stated previously, depression is common in HIV-positive patients and may be complicated by psychosis. The incidence of depression in AIDS patients is higher than in the general population. ECT has been useful in treating psychotically depressed patients with AIDS without reported adverse effects on memory. Mania in the HIV-positive population has been attributed to infection of the CNS or potential effects of antiviral drugs.

CHAPTER VI
PSYCHOTIC DISORDERS

Items 219-232

Choose the **BEST** response.

219. All the following symptoms are characteristic of psychosis **EXCEPT**:

    (A)   hallucinations
    (B)   delusions
    (C)   thought disorder
    (D)   ego-dystonic obsessions
    (E)   ideas of reference

220. Psychotic symptoms are among the core criteria for

    (A)   paranoid schizophrenia
    (B)   schizoid personality disorder
    (C)   schizoaffective disorder
    (D)   A and C only
    (E)   A, B, and C

221. Which of the following medical conditions may present with prominent psychotic symptoms?

    (A)   hypocalcemia
    (B)   hyperglycemia
    (C)   hypercholesterolemia
    (D)   A and C only
    (E)   A, B, and C

222. Other medical causes of psychotic symptoms include

    (A)   vitamin deficiency
    (B)   CNS infections
    (C)   sedative withdrawal
    (D)   A and C only
    (E)   A, B, and C

223. Delirium differs from schizophrenic psychosis in

    (A)   typical age of onset
    (B)   disrupting level of consciousness, orientation, and problem solving ability
    (C)   sudden rather than gradual onset
    (D)   A and C only
    (E)   A, B, and C

224. The "four As" of Eugen Bleuler's concept of schizophrenia include all of the following **EXCEPT**:

    (A)   animation
    (B)   ambivalence
    (C)   affective flattening
    (D)   autism
    (E)   associational disturbances

225. "Schneiderian symptoms"

    (A)   were described as features of schizophrenia by Kurt Schneider
    (B)   include so-called "ideas of reference"
    (C)   are also called "first rank symptoms"
    (D)   A and C only
    (E)   A, B, and C

226. All the following are classic ideas of reference **EXCEPT**:

    (A)   thought insertion, thought withdrawal
    (B)   thought broadcasting
    (C)   believing one is controlled by an outside force
    (D)   deriving idiosyncratic, personalized meaning from neutral or general stimuli
    (E)   believing one is related to famous people

227. Negative symptoms of schizophrenia include

    (A)   affective flattening
    (B)   avolition, apathy
    (C)   anhedonia/asociality
    (D)   A and C only
    (E)   A, B, and C

228. The **MOST** common hallucinations in schizophrenic psychoses are

   (A)   visual
   (B)   gustatory
   (C)   auditory
   (D)   tactile
   (E)   olfactory

229. A patient's belief that there is the plot to destroy the planet and that he is the chosen one to save it would be called

   (A)   hallucination
   (B)   illusion
   (C)   delusion
   (D)   idea of reference
   (E)   perseveration

230. The **MOST** common delusions in schizophrenic psychoses are

   (A)   delusions of bodily illness
   (B)   delusions of persecution
   (C)   delusional jealousy
   (D)   delusions of poverty
   (E)   None of the above

231. All of the following delusions are considered "mood congruent" in depression **EXCEPT**:

   (A)   hypochondriacal delusions
   (B)   delusions of guilt
   (C)   delusions of poverty
   (D)   bizarre delusions
   (E)   nihilistic delusions

232. The **MOST** common delusions in mania are

   (A)   bizarre delusions
   (B)   grandiose delusions
   (C)   belief that people have been replaced by impostors (Capgras's syndrome)
   (D)   delusions of external control
   (E)   delusions of time acceleration

ANSWERS AND TUTORIAL ON ITEMS 219-232

The answers are: **219-D; 220-D; 221-A; 222-E; 223-E; 224-A; 225-E; 226-E; 227-E; 228-C; 229-C; 230-B; 231-D; 232-B. Psychotic symptoms** are not extremes of the continuum of normal experience in the way that pathological moods (anxiety, depression) seem exaggerations of normal experience. Psychotic symptoms include hallucinations (perceptions of stimuli that are not there), delusions (false beliefs not shared by members of a cultural group), and thought disorder. Although schizophrenia is the prototypical psychotic disorder, psychotic symptoms also occur in other psychiatric disorders, especially extreme mania, severe depression, delirium and dementia. Although the neurological mechanisms that produce them are not well-understood, psychotic symptoms indicate a degree of brain dysfunction and serious illness. Being able to recognize and correctly classify them is an important medical diagnostic skill.

Clinically, schizophrenia is characterized by episodes of delusions, hallucinations, bizarre behavior, incoherent thought processes, and flat or inappropriate affect. It starts typically in early adolescence preceded by a prodrome of social withdrawal, unusual beliefs, and deterioration in hygiene and social or occupational functioning.

In Item 219, all the answers are typical **psychotic symptoms** except ego-dystonic obsessions. People with psychotic symptoms often lack insight into the unreality of their experience, that is, their symptoms are ego-syntonic. Ego-dystonic symptoms are those which patients recognize as irrational and abnormal, even if they cannot control them. Ego-dystonic obsessions are characteristic of **obsessive-compulsive disorder** (OCD); part of the anguish of patients with OCD derives from the awareness that their intrusive thoughts are senseless.

Schizoid personality disorder connotes a person who has little impulse towards involvement with others. Such people express little emotion, prefer solitary activities, are uninterested in sex, and seem cold and indifferent. The term schizoid was originally used to describe the premorbid personality of many schizophrenic patients, and these personality traits are often seen in that context. In DSM-IV, however, the criteria for schizoid personality disorder specifically exclude the psychotic manifestations of schizophrenia; by definition, the term refers to people who are schizoid without developing psychosis.

Psychotic symptoms can occur as manifestations of a variety of metabolic disturbances. Physicians must avoid dismissing someone with hallucinations or delusions as "merely psychotic;" psychotic symptoms in medically ill people indicate acute brain failure and may presage death. Psychotic symptoms can be manifestations of life-threatening chemical deficits; hypocalcemia (also hypomagnesemia, hyponatremia) are among the most threatening. High cholesterol is usually asymptomatic, and hyperglycemia (along with other excess metabolic states like hypercalcemia or hypernatremia) more often produces depression or sedation than psychosis. Other metabolic causes of psychotic symptoms include vitamin deficiencies (especially B_{12} and folate), endocrine imbalances (especially thyroid or corticosteroids), hypoxia, alcohol withdrawal, and various kinds of intoxication, including intoxication with prescribed drugs. In the past, CNS syphilis was a common cause of psychotic symptoms. In the age of AIDS, CNS infections are again important in the differential diagnosis of psychotic symptoms.

Delirium is a term which connotes a psychosis from serious bodily illness affecting the brain. By definition, it involves disruption of level of consciousness (indicating brainstem dysfunction). By contrast, simple problem solving ability, alertness and orientation are typically intact in schizophrenic psychoses. Being associated with severe illness, which rises with age, delirium is much more common in elderly patients. Idiopathic psychiatric disorders with psychotic symptoms (except depression with psychotic features) typically arise before age forty. Moreover, few organic causes of psychosis are relevant prior to age forty, with the exception of drug intoxication/withdrawal states, HIV invasion of the central nervous system, or CNS infections in AIDS. Delirium is typically of acute onset. Schizophrenia, by definition, has a gradual onset.

The current definition of **schizophrenia** derives from the work of three European psychiatrists: Emil Kraepelin, Eugen Bleuler, and Kurt Schneider. Bleuler, who practiced in a sanitarium where he saw patients in the chronic and residual phases of illness, emphasized the social withdrawal (autism), ambivalence, and loss of emotional expressiveness (affective flattening) of chronic patients. The associational disturbances he recognized included **thought disorder** and the fragmentation of mental functions, from which the term schizophrenia derives. Schneider's contribution was to highlight the acute psychotic symptoms, including delusions he called **ideas of reference** (thought insertion, thought deletion, thought broadcasting, special personalized meanings from neutral stimuli, external control of perceptions or behavior). Kraepelin, who preceded both Bleuler and Schneider, noted the relationship between the psychotic manifestations of the illness and the long-term deterioration of personality and functioning that accompany it. The current criteria for the disease embody all three facets, namely, positive psychotic symptoms (Schneider), negative symptoms (Bleuler) and chronicity (Kraepelin).

In evaluating patients with psychotic symptoms, it is helpful to know the characteristics of different types of psychosis. **Hallucinations,** sensory experiences without corresponding sensory stimulation, may occur in any sensory modality. Visual hallucinations are more common in delirium or psychedelic drug intoxication than in schizophrenia; olfactory and gustatory hallucinations are associated with partial complex seizures, and tactile hallucinations are characteristic of delirium tremens. Auditory hallucinations, especially intelligible voices commenting on the person's behavior as it occurs or making accusations, are the most common type in schizophrenia. However, hallucinations in other sensory modalities do occur during schizophrenic episodes, and auditory hallucinations occur in psychotic states other than schizophrenia. The presence or absence of one symptom or type of symptom does not determine the psychiatric diagnosis; diagnoses depend on patterns of symptoms and a characteristic course over time.

Delusions are fixed false beliefs. They are classified by their theme or content. **Grandiose delusions**, for example, are beliefs that a person possesses special powers. Persons who believe they are being persecuted, watched, or externally controlled are experiencing **paranoid delusions. Somatic delusions** are unusual beliefs about the functioning of the body.

Illusions are misinterpretations of existing sensory stimuli. When present, they suggest delirium or intoxication. Ideas of reference are defined above. **Perseveration** connotes persistent repetition of words, phrases, or simple motor behavior. It occurs in delirium or dementia as well as during psychosis of any cause.

Although the content of a particular delusion does not, by itself, prove the presence of one diagnosis or rule out another, different psychiatric disorders do have characteristic delusions.

Persecutory delusions are the most common form in both schizophrenia and delusional disorder. When delusions occur in association with a pathologic mood state, they may be consistent with the reported or observed mood (mood congruent) or inconsistent with it (mood incongruent). Mood congruent delusions appear to be markers of the severity of the mood disturbance; mood incongruent ones are less easily explained, but are known to confer a worse prognosis.

The characteristic **mood congruent delusions** of depression are beliefs that the person is ill or deteriorating (somatic), poor (poverty), guilty of some terrible sin, or the belief that the world is coming to an end (nihilistic). The most characteristic mood congruent manic delusion is belief that the person is special or has special powers (grandiose).

Items 233-237

Match a diagnosis in the answers below to the **MOST** appropriate clinical scenario in the items below. Answers may be used once, more than once, or not at all.

> (A)   Delusional disorder
> (B)   Schizotypal disorder
> (C)   Schizophreniform disorder
> (D)   Schizophrenia, paranoid type
> (E)   Schizophrenia, catatonic type
> (F)   Schizophrenia, disorganized type
> (G)   Schizophrenia, undifferentiated type
> (H)   Bipolar, manic, with mood congruent psychotic features
> (I)   Substance-induced psychosis
> (J)   Schizoaffective disorder
> (K)   Brief reactive psychosis

233.   Case I: A 22-year-old woman is brought in by her parents, for reasons she can't explain. On questioning, she does admit to hearing derogatory voices commenting on her every move for about the past week. She says she first felt not entirely herself about three months ago, just after graduating from college. She can't quite say how she felt unwell; things "just seemed different, somehow." She was planning to get a job, but has been staying at her parents' house, often sleeping much of the day and wandering at night. Her speech is a bit odd, with tangential answers to some questions. She has no relevant medical history. She has not smoked marijuana for two years and never used other drugs. She drinks only rarely on big social occasions.

234.   Case II: A 49-year-old woman complains to her primary care physician that she is under intolerable stress at work. Her manager seems to be trying to make her fail, and her coworkers treat her badly. She wonders whether they may be acting under the instructions of the FBI, who she believes have reams of files about her since she worked

for the Social Security Administration ten years ago. She has few friends, but she is close to her family and active in a hiking club. She feels discouraged and unhappy, though she enjoys her time away from work. Vegetative symptoms are limited to disrupted sleep on Mondays before work and some fatigue. She is overly talkative and circumstantial in trying to prove she is the target of investigation, but otherwise logical and coherent. She denies drug or alcohol use on the grounds that "You never know what someone might put into your drink."

235. Case III: A 50-year-old man is brought in by his wife because "He's going off again." She reports that he is not sleeping much, talks incessantly about plans to increase his business, and has run up unusual credit card debt from impulsive purchases. He is a social drinker, but lately he has been opening beers and leaving them around the house after only a few sips. He seems to be hearing voices, though he refuses to answers questions about this. His behavior includes starting tasks and not finishing them, eating furtively at odd times, rummaging in storage areas, and making lists. His wife reports his presentation is similar to an episode five years before. She thinks he has been hearing the voices for months, but his sleep changed only a week ago and he was acting fairly normally until three weeks ago.

236. Case IV: A 30-year-old man works as a custodian, though he has a college degree. He lives alone and has never had an intimate relationship. His chief complaint is that "I was told to come here." He says that he hears voices that tell him what is safe or not and what he should do. He admits to funny shock-like sensations in his body and says that "they" have planted electrical wires that cause him to have an orgasm or to experience pain anytime "they" want to. He smokes a joint of marijuana perhaps once every two months and drinks a few beers roughly as often. He presents himself in a stilted, robotic way, as though he were responding to military commands. He says he has had the shocks and heard the voices "for a long time" and was hospitalized when he told his family about them two years ago.

237. Case V: A 17-year-old high school student has been in and out of psychiatric treatment for five years. He was an isolated, quiet child. In adolescence, he gradually developed a thought disorder, keeping a detailed diary that is almost incoherent, filled with references to superheros and sports stars. His answers to questions are tangential, at times frankly illogical. He admits to auditory hallucinations. He smiles inappropriately and seems detached from his surroundings. He seems to lack awareness that anything is wrong. He also lacks initiative, though he will generally follow instructions to bathe, or put something away, or take his medicine.

ANSWERS AND TUTORIAL ON ITEMS 233-237

The answers are: **233-C; 234-A; 235-J; 236-D; 237-G**. In **case I**, the two main diagnoses to be considered are some form of **schizophrenia** or **schizophreniform disorder**. The patient has many schizophrenic symptoms, including disorganized behavior, decreased social and occupational functioning, auditory hallucinations and thought disorder. However, she does not meet the criterion for schizophrenia that symptoms, either psychotic, prodromal, or residual, be present for at least six months. This places her in the category of schizophreniform disorder.

In **case II**, the patient has classic **delusional disorder**, with nonbizarre delusions occurring in the absence of thought disorder, deterioration of social behavior, or extreme mood states. Being functionally intact and free of other psychotic symptoms distinguishes delusional disorder from schizophrenia. The absence of extreme moods rules out schizoaffective disorder.

In **case III**, the patient has both **manic symptoms** (expansiveness, decreased need for sleep, impulsivity, especially related to spending, loss of judgment, disorganized behavior) and psychotic symptoms (auditory hallucinations). His lack of insight is characteristic of either mania or psychosis. The need to get history from a third party is typical. What distinguishes this from schizophrenia is that the patient appears to have a fully developed abnormal mood state. What distinguishes it from bipolar disorder, manic, with mood congruent psychotic features, is that the psychotic symptoms were present for a long time prior to the onset of the affective ones. The patient's relatively intact social adaptation--he is married and employed--are consistent with schizoaffective disorder and would be unusual in schizophrenia. His disorganized behavior and vegetative signs rule out delusional disorder.

In **case IV**, the patient meets the criteria for **schizophrenia, paranoid type**. He has had symptoms for more than six months, he has more than one psychotic symptom (hallucinations and delusions, especially bizarre delusions [impossibilities, such as implantation of electrical wires without a person's knowledge]), and he is socially impaired, isolated and holding a job below his level of education. He does not have prominent mood symptoms, ruling out schizoaffective disorder, and his use of substances is far too little to account for his symptoms, ruling out psychosis secondary to substance abuse. The paranoid subclassification refers to the nature of his delusions and to his stilted, quasimilitary social behavior. Although impaired, he is independent and able to function on a day-to-day basis. Patients with paranoid type schizophrenia tend to be less impaired than those who are disorganized or catatonic. The different subtypes may, however, not represent valid distinctions. The same patient may meet criteria for different subtypes during different periods of exacerbation.

In **case V**, the patient has all the features of **undifferentiated schizophrenia**, including insidious onset, prominent thought disorder, hallucinations, marked functional impairment, and peculiar affect. The premorbid social isolation is typical, and the early age of onset is a bad prognostic sign.

Choose the **BEST** response.

238. Which of the following are **TRUE** statements concerning schizophrenia?

   (A) The condition can be reliably diagnosed cross-culturally using DSM-IV or other standardized criteria.
   (B) The general population prevalence of schizophrenia is roughly 1%.
   (C) Patients may have "soft" neurological signs, indicating subtle or diffuse brain dysfunction, though these are not always present.
   (D) A and C only.
   (E) A, B, and C

239. Neurological "soft signs" include

   (A) mixed dominance
   (B) inability to perceive two stimuli simultaneously
   (C) clumsiness, tremor, dysmetria
   (D) A and C only
   (E) A, B, and C

240. All the following statements are **TRUE** about the genetics of schizophrenia **EXCEPT**:

   (A) In a family with one schizophrenic parent, the risk of schizophrenia in a child is 5-6%.
   (B) Monozygotic twins show an 85% concordance for schizophrenia; in dizygotic twins, the concordance is 50%.
   (C) If both parents in a family have schizophrenia, the risk of schizophrenia in their offspring approaches 50%.
   (D) Adoption studies have shown that genetically at risk children adopted into normal families develop schizophrenia closer to the rate predicted by their genetic endowment than to the rate predicted by the rearing environment.
   (E) Neurodevelopmental trauma (complications of pregnancy or delivery, early CNS trauma or infections) enhances the risk that genetic vulnerability to schizophrenia will be expressed in clinical illness.

241. Which of the following statements **BEST** summarizes the contribution of family environment to the course of schizophrenia?

   (A)   Parents of schizophrenics create repeated double bind (no-win) situations that substantially contribute to the development of the disorder.
   (B)   High expressed emotion (hostility, nonacceptance of the legitimacy of the illness, and overinvolvement) contributes to the frequency and severity of relapses in established schizophrenia.
   (C)   Families of schizophrenics often seem detached or disengaged from one another and from the patient.
   (D)   Early loss of a parent from divorce or death appears to contribute to the development of schizophrenia.
   (E)   Return to the family environment after an acute episode is nearly always preferable to placement in a sheltered living situation and always preferable to placement in an independent living situation.

242. Good prognosis in schizophrenia is associated with

   (A)   acute onset
   (B)   mood-related symptoms
   (C)   absence of signs of neurological impairment
   (D)   A and C only
   (E)   A, B, and C

243. The "dopamine hypothesis," which posits overactivity of dopamine pathways in schizophrenia, is supported by

   (A)   the effectiveness of medications that block dopamine receptors
   (B)   the exacerbating effect of amphetamines on schizophrenic symptoms
   (C)   the finding of increased D_2 receptors in the caudate and nucleus accumbens regions in postmortem studies of schizophrenic brains
   (D)   A and C only
   (E)   A, B, and C

244. Dopamine pathways in the brain include

   (A)   mesolimbic tract
   (B)   corpus callosum
   (C)   nigrostriatal tract
   (D)   A and C only
   (E)   A, B, and C

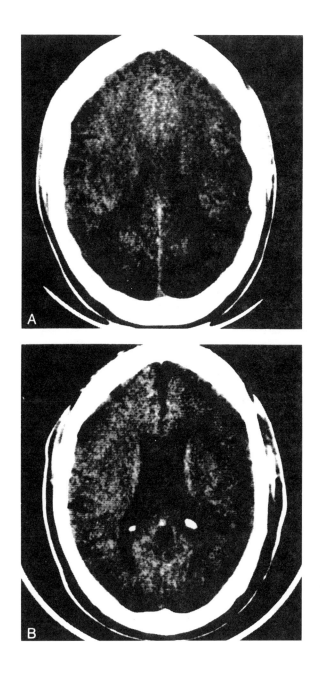

Figure 6.1

245. The relevant neuroanatomic finding shown by the CT scans in **Figure 6.1** of a normal and a schizophrenic brain is

    (A)   presence of narrowed lateral ventricles in the schizophrenic brain
    (B)   presence of enlarged lateral ventricles in the schizophrenic brain
    (C)   signs of diffuse microcalcification in the schizophrenic brain
    (D)   absence of any significant abnormality in either brain
    (E)   narrowing of sulci in the schizophrenic brain

246. Neurophysiologic abnormalities found using PET and SPECT in schizophrenia include

    (A)   evidence of generally decreased cerebral blood flow compared to controls
    (B)   decreased functional dopamine receptor binding activity in the striatum
    (C)   relative decrease in flood flow to the frontal lobes, consistent with evidence of defective ability to activate the prefrontal cortex
    (D)   A and C only
    (E)   A, B, and C

ANSWERS AND TUTORIAL ON ITEMS 238-246

The answers are: **238-E; 239-E; 240-B; 241-B; 242-E; 243-E; 244-D; 245-B; 246-C**. The **heterogeneity of schizophrenia** has presented a major challenge to medical research, resulting in a variety of explanatory hypotheses and controversies. Although European scientists in the late nineteenth and early twentieth centuries postulated a cryptic organic etiology, mid-century psychiatrists developed the argument that schizophrenia arose most frequently from social or environmental causes in people with otherwise normal brains. In recent decades, converging lines of research, including genetic-epidemiologic studies, neuroimaging, functional neuroimaging, and pharmacologic treatment studies, have supported a return to the presumption that schizophrenia (though not necessarily briefer psychotic conditions) typically results from organic brain dysfunction. These studies suggest the partial localization of schizophrenic brain dysfunction to the dopaminergic pathways of the brain, especially those involving the prefrontal cortex. However, a variety of other neurophysiologic abnormalities may also be involved in the pathogenesis of schizophrenia; indeed, as currently defined, schizophrenia is probably not a single disease but a family of related diseases, with different underlying mechanisms. Social environmental factors do affect the course of schizophrenia, and the possibility that social environmental factors alone may produce some cases of the disease cannot be dismissed based on current evidence.

All the answers in Item 238 are correct, and all support the likely link between organic dysfunction and schizophrenia. If the illness were induced by social/environmental factors, one would predict much higher rates in some cultures than in others, and the absence of the disease in cultures that lack the presumed causal factors. The presence of the same disease at roughly the same rate in different cultures thus supports causal biologic factors. Neurological soft signs include difficulty with spatial orientation, inability to simultaneously recognize multiple stimuli, poor coordination, pathological reflexes (frontal release signs), and incomplete lateralization. All are evidence of cortical or cerebellar brain dysfunction.

Studies that compare **concordance** for illness in monozygotic and dizygotic twins are a standard methodology for demonstrating the contribution of genetic factors to a condition. In a genetic illness such as sickle cell disease, concordance will approach 100% in monozygotic twins, who share all their genes. The concordance rate in dizygotic twins will be the same as for siblings if no environmental factor related to twinship is involved in the pathogenesis of the disease. In schizophrenia, the concordance rate in monozygotic twins (around 46%) is higher than the concordance rate in dizygotic twins (14%). Statement B incorrectly overstates the concordance rates in both cases. The near 50% monozygotic twin concordance rate and the higher concordance for monozygotic compared to dizygotic twins are consistent with a significant genetic contribution to the illness. These findings also imply that full expression of the disease may require nongenetic factors.

Family variables have been intensively studied as nongenetic factors that might cause schizophrenia. Many families with a schizophrenic member are disrupted by irresolvable conflicts, emotional dyscontrol, detached or overclose relationships, and the like. Such difficulties may stem from both the abnormal social behavior of members with schizophrenia or subtle social deficits in those with high genetic loading for the illness, and from the difficulty normal family members have in dealing with the behavior of a psychotic person. Adoption studies have demonstrated that family environment does not, by itself, cause schizophrenia. Adoptions studies show that children not biologically at risk for schizophrenia do not develop the illness when raised in dysfunctional adoptive families (including those with a schizophrenic member) while genetically at risk children develop schizophrenia even when raised in healthy families. However, family factors do play a role in the illness. Studies have repeatedly demonstrated increased rates of relapse and greater need for antipsychotic medication in patients who live in families where they are criticized and treated with hostility by an overinvolved relative, usually a parent. Thus, family variables are exacerbating rather than causal factors in schizophrenia.

Items 247-252

Parents bring their 19-year-old son to a physician for evaluation. They report that over the past few months their son has become socially isolated. He tends to stay in his room, refusing to bathe or go out with friends. He is suspicious about the intentions of others including his family, saying that they are trying to poison him out of envy. Recently he began to talk about the "plot to destroy the planet" and his special mission to save the world. Upon examination, he describes hearing voices of unknown people commenting about his behavior and giving him instructions on how to go about saving the world.

247. All of the following are possible diagnoses in this case **EXCEPT**:

   (A)   schizophrenia
   (B)   phencyclidine abuse
   (C)   bipolar disorder, manic phase, with psychotic features
   (D)   somatization disorder
   (E)   steroid psychosis

248. The medication that is **MOST** likely to relieve the auditory hallucinations of this patient is

   (A)   fluoxetine
   (B)   clozapine
   (C)   benztropine
   (D)   tranylcypromine
   (E)   lithium carbonate

249. Upon further evaluation you have made the diagnosis of schizophrenia. All of the following are **TRUE** statements about the prognosis in this condition **EXCEPT**:

   (A)   Acute psychotic symptoms usually remit, especially after the first episode.
   (B)   Schizophrenia is characterized by remissions and exacerbations with recovery after each episode being incomplete.
   (C)   Good prognosis is associated with the early onset of symptoms.
   (D)   Although about 30% of patients have a favorable course, the majority experience gradual deterioration in social and occupational functioning.
   (E)   Absence of positive family history for schizophrenia and the presence of mood symptoms warrant a good prognosis.

250. Life time prevalence of schizophrenia in the general population is

    (A)   0.5%
    (B)   3%
    (C)   over 5%
    (D)   about 1%
    (E)   difficult to estimate due to the diverse nature of symptomatology

251. All of the following are **TRUE** regarding etiologic factors that play a role in the development of schizophrenia **EXCEPT**:

    (A)   There is evidence for dopamine hyperactivity in the limbic system and dopamine deficiency in the striatum.
    (B)   Genetic studies of schizophrenia suggest an autosomal dominant transmission with variable penetrance.
    (C)   Typical age of onset after puberty and prior to age 45 indicate the presence of a neurodevelopmental defect.
    (D)   Family interactions marked by high levels of expressed hostile and critical emotions contribute to relapses in susceptible individuals but do not cause the illness.
    (E)   Slight increase in the incidence of schizophrenia in people born during winter months suggests possible viral etiology in some cases.

252. All of the following are among the criteria for the diagnosis of schizophrenia **EXCEPT**:

    (A)   grossly disorganized behavior
    (B)   duration of disturbance for no more than two weeks
    (C)   avolition
    (D)   delusions
    (E)   decline in social and occupational functioning

ANSWERS AND TUTORIAL ON ITEMS 247-252

The answers are: **247-D; 248-B; 249-C; 250-D; 251-B; 252-B. Somatization disorder** (D) is the only condition among those listed that is not associated with psychosis. It is characterized by excessive preoccupation with vague and numerous physical complaints for which there is no physiological basis. A paranoid psychosis may occur as part of schizophrenia, phencyclidine intoxication, steroid abuse or schizoaffective disorder.

The mainstay of the **treatment of schizophrenia** is **neuroleptic medication**. **Clozapine** (B) is a new neuroleptic agent. It is remarkable for its efficacy in treatment of drug-resistant patients and for lacking the extrapyramidal side-effects of typical neuroleptics. Clozapine, however, is associated with increased risk for seizures and agranulocytosis. Lithium carbonate has been used as a adjuvant drug, but by itself is not capable of ameliorating psychotic symptoms. Benztropine is an anticholinergic agent frequently used to counteract the extrapyramidal effects of typical neuroleptics. In large doses, it may decrease the efficacy of antipsychotic drugs.

The **course of schizophrenia** is characterized by slow deterioration with repeated episodes of psychosis. Early onset of illness (C), warrants poor prognosis. Although approximately 30% of the population with this illness has minimal impairment, the majority suffer the effects of chronic illness. Factors that predict a good outcome include negative family history of schizophrenia, **late** age of onset, good premorbid functioning, a precipitating event, the presence of a mood disturbance and an abundance of florid psychotic features such as delusions and hallucinations.

The **prevalence of schizophrenia** around the world is remarkably constant and is between one and two percent of the population (D). The prevalence is higher in some geographic regions, giving rise to the hypothesis of a viral etiology for this illness. While presenting with various symptoms, schizophrenia is a well-defined syndrome that can be studied epidemiologically.

The **etiology of schizophrenia** is largely unknown, although many theories exist. There is no hard evidence for the autosomal transmission of schizophrenia (B). The best understood genetic model of schizophrenia is that a gene or set of genes confers vulnerability to the disease and that phenotypic expression is brought on by stressors (social, biologic, or environmental). Genetic studies also show family clustering in this disease. Monozygotic twins have an increased concordance rate for the disease even if separated at birth and reared apart.

Other conditions present with schizophrenia-like aspects. Phencyclidine intoxication frequently presents with agitation and psychosis indistinguishable from schizophrenia though usually of shorter duration. Looking for the signs of delirium (especially nystagmus and autonomic signs) helps to differentiate the two. Psychosis resulting from the intake of steroids can also present similarly. Bipolar disorder, manic phase may be marked by agitation and grandiose delusions in addition to mood symptoms.

The DSM-IV criteria for the diagnosis of schizophrenia include the presence of delusions, prominent hallucinations, disorganized speech or behavior as well as negative symptoms such as alogia, avolition, and flattened affect. Two or more of these symptoms must be present for at least one month. Signs of the disorder, which may include subthreshold symptoms or functional impairment, must last at least 6 months. Deterioration in social and occupational functioning must occur. Other conditions, such as mood disorders and organic causes of psychosis, must be ruled out.

253. All of the following distinguish schizoaffective disorder, bipolar type, from schizophrenia, **EXCEPT**:

   (A)   severity of illness in the acute psychotic phase
   (B)   presence of prominent mood symptoms
   (C)   prognosis
   (D)   course of illness
   (E)   family history

254. The treatment regimen for schizoaffective disorder may include all of the following, **EXCEPT**:

   (A)   haloperidol
   (B)   psychotherapy
   (C)   lithium
   (D)   buspirone
   (E)   hospitalization

ANSWERS AND TUTORIAL ON ITEMS 253 AND 254

The answers are: **253-A; 254-D**. In many ways **schizoaffective disorder** has been a "wastebasket" diagnosis for conditions that do not readily fit criteria for schizophrenia or major mood disorders (major depression or bipolar disorders). It is distinguished from schizophrenia by the presence of **prominent** mood symptoms during the active phase of psychosis, somewhat better prognosis (especially in schizoaffective disorder, bipolar type), family history of mood disorders, nondeteriorating course and responsiveness to lithium.

Schizoaffective disorder, like many other psychotic disorders, is treated symptomatically. Thus, during the phase of psychosis, **neuroleptics** such as haloperidol are useful. Lithium is indicated if manic symptoms are prominent and as an adjunct to neuroleptics. Hospitalization is often necessary to prevent harm to self and others.

Psychotherapy, especially of supportive type, must be part of the management of any chronic mental disorder. Buspirone is an anxiolytic used largely for the treatment of generalized anxiety disorder and is not particularly useful in management of schizoaffective disorder, bipolar type.

Items 255-259

Choose the **BEST** response.

        (A)   Schizoaffective disorder
        (B)   Bipolar disorder
        (C)   Both
        (D)   Neither

255.   Grandiose delusions may constitute a central feature of the clinical presentation.

256.   Depression is common and can be treated with standard antidepressants.

257.   Requires a two week period of delusions or hallucinations in the absence of mood symptoms.

258.   Females are 5 times more affected than males.

259.   Hallucinations are a frequent cause of this condition.

ANSWERS AND TUTORIAL ON ITEMS 255-259

The answers are: **255-C; 256-C; 257-A; 258-D; 259-D. Grandiose delusions** are a sign of psychosis and are not specific for any psychotic disorder. They can be present in schizoaffective disorder, schizophrenia, bipolar disorder or delusional disorder.

    Depression is a common syndrome in bipolar disorder and may be present in schizoaffective disorder, depressed type. It is usually treated with standard antidepressant medication. Neuroleptics or lithium may also be required to forestall antidepressant induced mania.

    The definition of **schizoaffective disorder** requires a two week period of psychosis in the absence of mood symptoms. In bipolar disorder, if psychosis is present it occurs in the context of prominent mood symptoms.

    Bipolar disorder occurs with approximately equal frequency in either sex and the incidence of schizoaffective disorder is only slightly greater in females.

    While **hallucinations** may be prominent in either disorder, they are a symptom and not an etiologic agent.

Items 260-267

Choose the **BEST** response.

260. Indications for the use of antipsychotic agents include all of the following **EXCEPT**:

   (A)   bipolar disorder, manic phase
   (B)   schizoaffective disorder
   (C)   delirium with agitation
   (D)   panic disorder with agoraphobia
   (E)   major depression with mood congruent delusions

261. All of the following are adverse effects associated with some typical antipsychotic agents **EXCEPT**:

   (A)   akathisia
   (B)   pigmentation retinopathy
   (C)   hypertension
   (D)   dry mouth
   (E)   tardive dyskinesia

Items 262-267

Match each of the following drugs with the **MOST** likely common side-effects in the items below. Answers may be used once, more than once, or not at all.

   (A)   Phenelzine
   (B)   Thioridazine
   (C)   Fluoxetine
   (D)   Amitriptyline
   (E)   Nortriptyline
   (F)   Lithium
   (G)   Methylphenidate
   (H)   Fluphenazine
   (I)   Trazodone

262. Doses exceeding 800 mg/day may cause retinal pigment deposition frequently resulting in blindness.

263. On rare occasions, has been known to cause priapism.

264. A tricyclic antidepressant preferentially used in elderly patients due to minimal effects on orthostatic blood pressure.

265. Can lead to severe hypertensive crisis and subarachnoid hemorrhage when taken with aged cheeses or wine.

266. Diabetes insipidus is a rare but important adverse effect of this agent.

267. Transient growth suppression, anorexia, and insomnia are the main adverse effects of this drug used in the treatment of depression and attention-deficit/hyperactivity disorder.

ANSWERS AND TUTORIALS ON ITEMS 260-267

The answers are: **260-D; 261-C; 262-B; 263-I; 264-E; 265-A; 266-F; 267-G**. Antipsychotic medications are not specific for any particular disorder but are used to treat severe agitation, delusions, hallucinations, and any other symptoms of psychosis. **Panic disorder with agoraphobia** (D) is an anxiety disorder characterized by intense fear of death or "going crazy" accompanied by somatic symptoms of autonomic arousal such as sweating, trembling, diarrhea, shortness of breath and palpitations. Agoraphobia is a fear of being in a place where panic symptoms might cause problems or help might be unavailable. No psychotic symptoms are associated with panic disorder. Treatment generally consists of benzodiazepines, antidepressants, and cognitive-behavioral therapy.

The **side-effects** of the typical **neuroleptics** relate to the potency of given compounds. Thus, high potency agents such as **haloperidol** are associated with extrapyramidal symptoms including acute dystonias, akathisia, and pseudoparkinsonism. Low potency antipsychotic drugs such as **chlorpromazine** are commonly associated with sedation and anticholinergic side-effects, including blurred vision, constipation, and urinary retention. Presynaptic alpha blockade leads to **postural hypotension**, most prominently in low potency agents.

Side-effects that are specific to particular compounds include **pigmentation retinopathy** associated with daily intake of **thioridazine** in excess of 800 mg and grey skin discoloration and photosensitivity found with high doses of chlorpromazine. All neuroleptics can cause endocrine abnormalities such as weight gain, loss of sexual interest, galactorrhea, and gynecomastia. In addition, all typical neuroleptics can lead to **tardive dyskinesia**, a chronic movement disorder, after many years of use.

Although many neurotransmitter systems are affected by neuroleptics, the most commonly postulated mode of action is the blockade of **postsynaptic dopamine (D$_2$) receptors** in the nigrostriatal, mesolimbic, and tubuloinfundibular pathways. These pathways subserve movement, emotion/ideation, and prolactin secretion, accounting for the side-effects seen.

Clozapine, which is an atypical antipsychotic agent recently approved for use by the FDA, differs from older agents in that it does not produce significant extrapyramidal side-effects and has not been associated thus far with **tardive dyskinesia**.

Clozapine is not a phenothiazine. Among its properties are severe sedation due to histaminergic blockade, hypotension, anticholinergic side-effects, an increased risk for seizures and agranulocytosis. It is thought to be a stronger D_1 antagonist and to have prominent effect on serotonin transmission.

Antipsychotic agents are relatively safe drugs as a class. Overdoses of several grams of these drugs are frequently without sequelae. However, those agents with high anticholinergic properties are likely to exacerbate delirium, worsen glaucoma leading to acute angle closure, and worsen the course of phencyclidine intoxication secondary to the additive anticholinergic effects.

Phenelzine (A) is a **monamine oxidase inhibitor** (MAOI) used treating depression, bipolar disorder, and panic disorder. Overdoses of MAOIs lead to profound hypotension. When MAOIs are taken with **tyramine**-containing foods such as aged cheese, red wine, and pickled meats, hypertensive crises can occur because MAO is unavailable to metabolize tyramine. Chlorpromazine has been used to lower blood pressure during hypertensive crises resulting from MAOI/tyramine interaction.

Thioridazine (B) is a low potency neuroleptic that may cause ventricular arrhythmias when taken in overdose.

Fluoxetine (C) is a serotonin-specific reuptake inhibitor (SSRI) used to treat depression, obsessive-compulsive disorder, and anxiety disorders. It has virtually no cardiac side-effects, alpha-blocking properties, or anticholinergic side-effects. However, the half-life of its active metabolite is about 100 hrs. This makes the drug unsuitable for the treatment of frail, geriatric patients.

Amitriptyline (D) and **nortriptyline** (E) are both tricyclic antidepressants. Amitriptyline is a secondary amine which has potent anticholinergic, histaminergic, and alpha-blocking properties. It has been known to precipitate delirium in the elderly and in patients with organic impairments of the brain. Nortriptyline is a tertiary amine with low anticholinergic and alpha-blocking properties, making it a particularly suitable antidepressant in elderly patients prone to falls and confusion.

Lithium (F) salts are used in the treatment of bipolar disorder. While lithium revolutionized the treatment of manic depression, it is associated with serious toxic effects at doses only slightly higher than those required to treat manic symptoms. Thus, it has a narrow "therapeutic window". Short-term toxic effects include nausea, diarrhea, tremor, skin eruptions, and, occasionally, delirium. Long-term toxicity, even at therapeutic dosages, includes hypothyroidism, a rare form of interstitial nephritis, and diabetes insipidus.

Methylphenidate (G) is a stimulant related to amphetamine. It is most commonly used in the treatment of attention-deficit/hyperactivity disorder (ADHD) and certain types of depression in elderly and medically ill patients. Acute administration causes appetite suppression and insomnia. Some studies have shown transient growth suppression in children receiving methylphenidate.

Fluphenazine (H) is a high potency phenothiazine neuroleptic which is used in the treatment of psychosis. It is one of two neuroleptics currently available in depot form, allowing for biweekly maintenance therapy.

Trazodone (I) is an atypical antidepressant which does not have the major cardiac side-effects of tricyclics. It is frequently used as a hypnotic due to its lack of abuse potential. It is associated rarely with cases of priapism.

Items 268-272

Choose the **BEST** response.

268. All of the following are **TRUE** of the neuroleptic malignant syndrome (NMS) **EXCEPT**:

    (A)   It is similar in clinical presentation to malignant hyperthermia associated with the use of general anesthetics.
    (B)   Like malignant hyperthermia, NMS recurs upon subsequent administration of neuroleptics.
    (C)   Among the laboratory findings, leukocytosis, myoglobinuria, and a highly elevated muscle fraction of creatinine phosphokinase (CPK) are common.
    (D)   Major complications include acute renal failure, rhabdomyolysis, and cardiovascular collapse.
    (E)   NMS is an idiosyncratic reaction to the administration of most common neuroleptics, and can be life-threatening.

269. Which of the following is **TRUE** regarding NMS?

    (A)   It is associated only with the use of high potency neuroleptics.
    (B)   Once it occurs, the chance of survival is minimal.
    (C)   The best treatment is a switch to a lower potency neuroleptic.
    (D)   It has been reported with all known neuroleptics.
    (E)   No cases have been associated with the use of clozapine.

270. The management of NMS must include all the following **EXCEPT**:

    (A)   institution of supportive measures, such as intravenous hydration
    (B)   immediate discontinuation of the neuroleptic
    (C)   administration of intravenous mannitol
    (D)   frequent monitoring of vital signs
    (E)   administration of dantrolene sodium or bromocriptine

271. Choose the **BEST** description of the clinical presentation of NMS.

(A) Confusion, agitation, elevated temperature, blood pressure and pulse; muscle rigidity, akinesis and mutism.

(B) Agitation, low blood pressure and pulse, high temperature, paralysis and mutism.

(C) Clear sensorium, abnormal involuntary movements, elevated pulse, temperature and blood pressure.

(D) Sudden painful muscle contractions in the neck region.

(E) Mutism, flaccid paralysis, waxy flexibility, autonomic instability.

272. The **MOST** significant risk factors associated with the development of NMS are

(A) being male and young

(B) being female and young

(C) being male and old

(D) being female and old

(E) sex and age are not risk factors for the development of NMS

ANSWERS AND TUTORIAL ON ITEMS 268-272

The answers are: **268-B; 269-D; 270-C; 271-A; 272-A. Neuroleptic malignant syndrome** (NMS) is a rare, life-threatening complication of the use of antipsychotic medications. It has been reported with all known neuroleptics, including the atypical ones like clozapine. The use of high potency neuroleptics slightly increases the chance of developing NMS. The pathophysiology of NMS is unknown. It is thought to be related to the malignant hyperthermia which occasionally occurs with the use of general anesthetics. Unlike malignant hyperthermia, NMS is an idiosyncratic reaction which is unlikely to recur if the patient is rechallenged with the same neuroleptic in the future. Although many studies demonstrate the safety of rechallenging the patient with the same neuroleptic or a neuroleptic of similar class two weeks after the resolution of NMS, prudence dictates the choice of a low potency antipsychotic or clozapine. Clinically, the syndrome usually develops in the first two weeks of neuroleptic treatment. It is characterized by mental confusion, agitation, muscle rigidity, akinesis, and mutism. Associated symptoms include fever, frequently up to 107°F, sweating, elevated blood pressure and pulse. Laboratory findings include elevated white cell count, highly elevated MM fraction of creatinine phosphokinase, elevated liver enzymes, myoglobinuria and increased serum myoglobin. Complications are usually due to the rapid destruction of muscle tissue (rhabdomyolysis), acute renal failure due to blockade of the renal tubules by myoglobin, and cardiovascular collapse. While generally reversible, NMS has proven fatal in 20-30% of patients following the use of depot neuroleptics. Clinical management involves awareness of the syndrome, which leads to early diagnosis, and largely supportive measures directed at cooling the patient, maintaining normal blood pressure and pulse, and aggressive hydration to prevent damage to the renal tubules. Medication, when used, includes dantrolene sodium, bromocriptine, and, less commonly, amantadine.

Items 273-275

Choose the **BEST** response.

273. Which of the following statements are **TRUE** regarding the properties of atypical neuroleptics?

    (A)   They have antipsychotic efficacy with minimal extrapyramidal side-effects.
    (B)   They cause minimal prolactin elevation.
    (C)   They do not cause tardive dyskinesia.
    (D)   They are effective in treating negative symptoms of schizophrenia.
    (E)   All of the above

274. All of the following are atypical neuroleptics **EXCEPT**:

    (A)   olanzapine
    (B)   risperidone
    (C)   clozapine
    (D)   chlorpromazine
    (E)   sertindole

275. Pharmacological characteristics of the atypical neuroleptics, which may be responsible for their **UNIQUE** action are

    (A)   greater blockade of D_2 receptors than D_1 ones
    (B)   low level of activity at central muscarinic receptors
    (C)   high degree of blockade of serotonin $5\text{-}HT_{2A}$ receptors
    (D)   blockade of $alpha_1$ adrenoreceptors
    (E)   blockade of histamine H_1 receptors

ANSWERS AND TUTORIAL ON ITEMS 273-275

The answers are: **273-E; 274-D; 275-C**. The advent of a new class of antipsychotic medications, the **atypical neuroleptics**, has revolutionized the management of schizophrenia in the way that the discovery of chlorpromazine marked a new era in the treatment of psychosis. The atypical agents are a chemically heterogeneous group of compounds that share several clinical and pharmacological characteristics. Most atypical neuroleptics ameliorate the negative as well as positive symptoms of schizophrenia. They have not yet been found to cause tardive dyskinesia and have minimal extrapyramidal side-effects. In causing minimal prolactin elevation, these compounds are less likely than typical neuroleptics to produce sexual dysfunction, gynecomastia, and galactorrhea.

The ability of these drugs to treat the **negative symptoms** of schizophrenia is believed to be due to their ability to block reuptake of serotonin at the 5-HT_{2A} receptor. The extent of this blockade varies among different compounds, with sertindole and risperidone being the most potent 5-HT_{2A} blockers, clozapine exhibiting an intermediate degree of blockade, and olanzapine being the weakest among the atypical neuroleptics in its ability to block serotonin reuptake. It is important to note that while 5-HT_{2A} blockade is found in all atypical compounds, chlorpromazine, the prototypical neuroleptic, is also a potent inhibitor of the reuptake of serotonin. Thus, activity at the 5-HT_{2A} receptor is, perhaps, a necessary but not sufficient condition for the compound to exhibit atypical properties.

Most typical neuroleptics have greater activity at D_2 receptors than D_1 receptors. It takes approximately 70% occupancy of D_2 receptor sites for a compound to have antipsychotic properties. At occupancies significantly higher than 70%, extrapyramidal side- effects become manifest. It is the balance between D_2 blockade and 5-HT_{2A} blockade that accounts for the low extrapyramidal side-effect profile of the atypical neuroleptics.

All neuroleptics are potent $alpha_1$ blockers, leading to postural hypotension associated with their use. A high degree of antimuscarinic activity correlates with low incidence of extrapyramidal side-effects and may be present in both typical and atypical neuroleptics.

Items 276-281

Match the drug in the answers below with the **MOST** appropriate description of its side- effects or modes of action in the items. Answers may be used once, more than once, or not at all.

(A) Risperidone
(B) Venlafaxine
(C) Chlorpromazine
(D) Clozapine
(E) Clonazepam
(F) Phenelzine
(G) Olanzapine
(H) Amitriptyline

276. Increased incidence of agranulocytosis delayed the marketing of this drug and has limited its use despite demonstrated efficacy in the treatment of the negative symptoms of schizophrenia.

277. While structurally and pharmacologically similar to clozapine, this drug is characterized by decreased incidence of seizures.

278. This drug has strong activity at dopamine D_2 and serotonin $5\text{-}HT_{2A}$ receptors, blocking both, which accounts for its efficacy for both the positive and negative symptoms of schizophrenia.

279. Tardive dyskinesia occurs after long-term use of this drug, and may not be reversible upon discontinuation of its use.

280. Sialorrhea, which can be quite bothersome, is a unique side-effect of this drug, despite its strong anticholinergic properties.

281. This drug is used for the management of bipolar disorder, epilepsy, and as an adjuvant treatment of psychosis.

ANSWERS AND TUTORIAL ON ITEMS 276-281

The answers are: **276-D; 277-G; 278-A; 279-C; 280-D; 281-E. Clozapine** (D), when it first appeared on the market, showed great promise in the management of treatment resistant schizophrenia. Unfortunately, it was recalled in 1975 due to an alarming incidence of agranulocytosis, with a high number of fatal outcomes. While the average incidence of agranulocytosis associated with the use of neuroleptics is 0.04%-0.5%, it rises to 1-2% with clozapine. The drug was reintroduced in 1990, with strict guidelines for weekly monitoring of white cell counts and absolute neutrophil counts. If a patient develops leukopenia while on clozapine, the drug is immediately discontinued and the patient should never be rechallenged with it. Among the other side-effects of this drug are significantly increased incidence of seizures and sialorrhea. It is of particular interest that clozapine leads to hypersalivation, even though it is a highly anticholinergic compound. It has been shown that while inhibiting some muscarinic receptors, clozapine actually acts as an agonist at other muscarinic sites.

Olanzapine (G) is closely related to clozapine. It differs in that it does not cause agranulocytosis and is not associated with any increased incidence of seizures. Olanzapine is sedating and may lead to orthostatic changes and weight gain.

Risperidone (A) is an atypical neuroleptic, effective for both positive and negative symptoms in schizophrenia. It tends to cause more extrapyramidal side-effects than clozapine, but is less sedating and better tolerated. It owes its profile to a strong D_2 and 5-HT_{2A} blockade. It does not increase the risk of agranulocytosis or seizures, but it may cause restlessness and agitation.

Chlorpromazine (C) has been associated, as all other typical neuroleptics, with the development of tardive dyskinesia after long-term use.

Clonazepam (E) is a benzodiazepine. It has a long half-life, which makes it ideal for the management of withdrawal states. It is also an anticonvulsant. Used in addition to lithium, carbamazepine, valproate, and neuroleptics, it is useful in the management of acute mania. It has also been used to treat anxiety disorder and panic attacks.

Items 282-287

Choose the **BEST** response.

282.   Tardive dyskinesia (TD) is a condition resulting from

     (A)   traumatic hemisection of the spinal cord
     (B)   sequelae of Parkinson's disease
     (C)   parasitic infection of the caudate nucleus
     (D)   long-term use of conventional neuroleptics
     (E)   effects of Wilson's disease on the brain

283. The **BEST** definition of TD is

(A) involuntary, tonic-clonic movements of the extremities
(B) involuntary, purposeless choreoathetoid movements of orofacial area, extremities, and the trunk
(C) abnormal movement disorder, which appears in Stage 4 sleep
(D) a movement disorder associated with the use of minor tranquilizers
(E) None of the above.

284. The abnormal involuntary movements of TD

(A) may be volitionally suppressed, at least temporarily
(B) are exacerbated by stress
(C) are absent during sleep
(D) A and C only
(E) A, B, and C

285. All of the following are **TRUE** regarding TD **EXCEPT**:

(A) 4-7% of the elderly develop TD in the absence of exposure to neuroleptics.
(B) Temporary discontinuation of neuroleptic use will exacerbate the symptoms of TD.
(C) Increase in the dose of neuroleptic will mask the symptoms of TD.
(D) The prevalence of TD in the psychiatric population is as high as 70%.
(E) Prevalence of up to 30% was reported in schizophrenic populations prior to advent of antipsychotic medication.

286. The risk factors for development of TD are

(A) advanced age
(B) drug dose
(C) female sex
(D) All of the above
(E) None of the above

287. All of the following are appropriate steps in the management of TD **EXCEPT**:

(A) switching to a higher potency neuroleptic
(B) switching to clozapine
(C) initiating vitamin E therapy
(D) starting a trial of clonazepam
(E) discontinuing the neuroleptic

ANSWERS AND TUTORIAL ON ITEMS 282-287

The answers are: **282-D; 283-B; 284-E; 285-D; 286-D; 287-A**. **Tardive dyskinesia** (TD) is a movement disorder most commonly associated with the **long-term use of neuroleptics**. It presents itself with abnormal, purposeless, involuntary movements, usually of choreoathetoid nature, involving the orofacial area, extremities and trunk. The area most commonly involved is the mouth, with tongue darting and lip smacking. Facial mannerisms are also common. Rare forms of TD involve the muscles of trunk and diaphragm, severely interfering with breathing and ambulating.

The range of the disorder spans between cosmetic disfigurement and life-threatening impairments. While most commonly associated with the use of neuroleptics, it is noteworthy that TD existed at a prevalence rate of about 20-30% in the general schizophrenic population prior to the advent of antipsychotic medications. Moreover, TD occurs in 4-7% of elderly people in the absence of any exposure to neuroleptics. TD is difficult to diagnose, especially in its milder form, because it is similar to mannerisms and stereotypies commonly found among schizophrenics. Other movement disorders, such as Wilson's disease, Parkinson's disease, and Sydenham's chorea must be ruled out.

The abnormal movements of TD, while involuntary, may be volitionally temporarily suppressed. They disappear in sleep and worsen with stress. The pathophysiology of TD is not fully understood. The prevailing theories include hypersensitivity of postsynaptic dopamine receptors after long-term blockade by neuroleptics. This hypothesis, while not particularly substantiated by anatomical and neuroimaging findings, accounts for the suppression of TD symptoms by transiently increasing the patient's neuroleptic and worsening of the symptoms if the neuroleptic is decreased. Other explanations include the possible formation of free radicals by antipsychotic medication leading to neuronal damage. Vitamin E and other antioxidant therapy has been found helpful in the management of TD. Finally, there is a hypothesis that a deficit in GABAergic transmission is responsible for the symptoms of TD. The use of **clonazepam**, a GABA agonist, has been helpful in treatment of this disorder. The risk factors for development of TD relate to the patient's age and the doses of neuroleptic used. Women seem to be also at an increased risk. The presence of mood symptoms in psychosis may also predispose one to later development of TD.

The management of this condition includes use of the minimal effective dose of neuroleptic, discontinuation of the offending drug upon emergence of symptoms, switching to clozapine, and using clonazepam and vitamin E.

CHAPTER VII
MOOD DISORDERS

Items 288-293

Choose the **BEST** response.

288. A major depressive episode differs from normal sadness in

    (A) including marked changes in vegetative functioning
    (B) being more severe and persistent
    (C) causing significant functional impairment
    (D) A and C only
    (E) A, B, and C

289. A depressive episode typically includes all the following symptoms **EXCEPT**:

    (A) insomnia
    (B) ideas of worthlessness/helplessness
    (C) negative view of the future
    (D) feelings of disgust or revulsion
    (E) diminished capacity for pleasure

290. By definition, a major depressive episode involves

    (A) at least a week of symptoms
    (B) seven of nine criterion symptoms
    (C) absence of an identifiable precipitant
    (D) All of the above
    (E) None of the above

291. Recognized symptom **PATTERNS** in depression include

    (A) increased sleep, psychomotor retardation, weight gain
    (B) decreased sleep, diurnal variation (mornings worse), anhedonia
    (C) decreased sleep, agitation, weight loss
    (D) A and C only
    (E) A, B, and C

292. Characteristic ("mood congruent") delusions in depression include

    (A)   delusions of poverty
    (B)   delusions of special powers
    (C)   delusions of external control
    (D)   A and C only
    (E)   A, B, and C

293. Mood congruent psychotic symptoms

    (A)   help differentiate depression with psychotic features from depression occurring secondary to schizophrenia
    (B)   signify a better prognosis than mood incongruent symptoms
    (C)   signify a worse prognosis than depression without any psychotic features
    (D)   All of the above
    (E)   None of the above

Items 294-301

Match the psychiatric conditions in the following list of answers below with the **MOST** appropriate clinical scenario in the items. Answers may be used once, more than once, or not at all.

    (A)   Major depressive episode
    (B)   Dysthymic disorder
    (C)   Major depressive episode with mood congruent psychotic features
    (D)   Major depressive episode with mood incongruent psychotic features
    (E)   Schizoaffective, depressed
    (F)   Bipolar disorder, most recent episode depressed
    (G)   Major depressive episode, melancholic
    (H)   Major depressive episode with atypical features
    (I)   Substance induced mood disorder
    (J)   Adjustment disorder with depressed mood
    (K)   Normal bereavement

294. **Patient I**. A 50-year-old woman is admitted to the hospital for the sixth time. She is withdrawn, irritable, fearful and restless. She reports feeling depressed for about six weeks, with difficulty falling and staying asleep and a fifteen pound weight loss due to loss of appetite. She has suicidal ideation with a plan to take an overdose, which she has done in the past under the influence of command auditory hallucinations. She hears

voices pretty much continuously, but when she is not depressed, they do not talk of suicide. She has been divorced for many years and has trouble holding jobs due to her suspiciousness and odd responses to other people.

295. **Patient II**. A 35-year-old woman wants her primary care physician to evaluate her for chronic fatigue syndrome. She does not have a history of viral or flu-like symptoms, just intense fatigue, hypersomnia (sleeping up to 11 hours a night), 10 lb weight gain, and generally low mood. She says she can feel better briefly when out with friends, but mostly she feels sad, discouraged to the point of hopelessness about becoming her normal self again, and worthless, because she is not the person she wants to be. While she says she would not intentionally hurt herself, she would be glad to "just disappear," if she could. She drinks socially, up to 2 beers every other weekend.

296. **Patient III**. A 50-year-old man feels sad and confused since being laid off from his job two months ago. He can't seem to get himself to look aggressively for another one, saying he is too old and no one will hire him. He sleeps normally, except on the nights before job interviews, but he feels tired and dragged down many days. He drinks a beer with dinner every third night. Occasionally, he has bouts of restlessness and pacing, though he does not describe full panic attacks. He has some thoughts that life is not worth living, but none of hurting himself.

297. **Patient IV**. A 64-year-old woman describes a five month history of depressed mood, markedly decreased sleep due to early morning awakening, 20 pound weight loss, crying spells and intensifying suicidal ideation. She says mornings are the hardest time, she feels so guilty about not getting up and doing all the things she should. After grieving the loss of her husband, who died three years ago, she became active in church groups and volunteer work. Now she just goes to work and comes home, since nothing feels worthwhile or enjoyable. She denies alcohol use and has no major medical problems except hypercholesterolemia managed with diet.

298. Medical evaluation of the symptoms of **patient IV** should include

    (A)   thyroid function tests
    (B)   LH; FSH
    (C)   4 PM cortisol
    (D)   A and C only
    (E)   A, B, and C

299. **Patient V**. A 20-year-old man comes to the college counselling service because he wants to feel happier. He says he has always been a "down kind of guy." He reports he finds it hard to make decisions, and that after he does, if something seems difficult, he gives up easily, since he can't believe it could work out. He has no idea what to do when he leaves college--nothing seems really appealing or possible to him. He often "forgets to eat" and tends to lose a little weight during the semester, regaining it when he is home.

His mood may brighten for a day or half a day, but always drops back quickly. He drinks on weekends, up to four or five beers with friends, but he says his mood is the same even during times when he doesn't go out drinking for months at a time.

300. **Patient VI.** A 60-year-old woman is brought in by her family for hoarding and refusing to spend even minimal amounts of money on necessities. She is convinced that she is on the verge of bankruptcy, which her family denies. She admits to hearing voices accusing her of having done awful things. She has not been able to sleep for more than five hours at a stretch for three months. She has lost almost ten pounds, and at night she paces, cries and wrings her hands for hours. The family reports that she is very different from her normal self--a quiet, but responsive and pleasant person. She did have a "nervous breakdown" in her mid-forties, from which she recovered fully after electroconvulsive treatment.

301. Which of the patients above is **MOST** likely to also have a seasonal pattern or nonpsychotic manic or hypomanic episodes?

    (A)   I
    (B)   II
    (C)   III
    (D)   IV
    (E)   V
    (F)   VI

ANSWERS AND TUTORIAL ON ITEMS 288-301

The answers are: **288-E; 289-D; 290-E; 291-E; 292-A; 293-D; 294-E; 295-H; 296-J; 297-G; 298-A; 299-B; 300-C; 301-B**. **Depression** as a psychiatric *symptom* exists partly on a continuum with normal reactions to loss, disappointment, frustration, or rejection. It may differ from a normal mood only in being unduly persistent or severe, as when acute symptoms last for years following bereavement. Sometimes, depressed mood is qualitatively different from grief or sadness. People may describe themselves as empty or anguished rather than merely sad. Patients may also have psychotic symptoms--especially critical hallucinations and delusions--when they are clinically depressed.

Because of the overlap with normal, the definition of depression as a *disorder* requires drawing an arbitrary line between illness and nonillness. By definition, a **major depressive episode** involves mood symptoms for at least **two weeks**, concurrent with **neurovegetative changes** in sleep, appetite, energy, capacity to experience pleasure, concentration, and motor behavior. In addition, depression involves characteristic beliefs or ideas, especially inappropriate guilt, thoughts of death or suicide, worthlessness, helplessness, loss of interest (apathy), and hopelessness. As defined in DSM-IV, a person needs five of the nine characteristic symptoms and one must be sadness or loss of interest or the capacity to experience pleasure (anhedonia). Disgust or revulsion, though clearly negative affects, are not among the criteria for depression.

As defined, the syndrome of depression is quite heterogeneous: people may sleep too little or too much, may gain or lose weight, may be retarded or agitated, have mostly ideational or mostly neurovegetative signs, and so on. Some of the different symptoms form characteristic patterns recognized as subtypes, to be covered below.

When **psychotic symptoms** occur in the context of a depressive episode, the distinction between mood congruent and mood incongruent delusions or hallucinations is a meaningful one. Mood congruent delusions, which include hypochondriacal beliefs, guilt, and nihilism in addition to delusions of poverty, are associated with a better prognosis than bizarre or incongruent ones. Psychotically depressed patients may also hear critical or derogatory voices.

Although **mood congruent symptoms** are less ominous than mood incongruent ones, any psychotic symptom in depression negatively affects outcome (and complicates treatment, see below). While the presence of psychotic symptoms does not require that a person be diagnosed with two disorders, at times that may be indicated. People with schizophrenia, for example, frequently experience depressive symptoms and sometimes have depressive episodes. In well-established schizophrenia, subthreshold levels of depressive symptoms are considered a part of the primary disorder. **Depressive episodes** in the course of **schizophrenia** may prompt a diagnosis of **schizoaffective disorder**, which requires that the psychotic symptoms persist during some phase when the mood symptoms have abated. Younger depressed patients with psychotic symptoms may turn out to be bipolar. In older patients, the presence of psychotic symptoms should prompt evaluation for delirium or dementia. Schizophrenia, schizoaffective disorder, bipolar disorder, and delirium/dementia all confer a worse prognosis than depression alone.

Patient I has **schizoaffective disorder**. She has a clear depressive syndrome, but by history she also has psychotic symptoms when not depressed. If she hallucinated only in close proximity to her depressive episodes, she would be classifiable as having major depressive episode with mood congruent psychotic features. Her poor social functioning is also more typical of a major psychotic disorder than of a mood disorder (though people with mood disorders often have social impairments that persist between episodes).

Patient II has **major depression with atypical features**, specifically hypersomnia, weight gain, psychomotor retardation, and preserved capacity for pleasure, despite a lack of initiative. Bipolar and bipolar II patients often have atypical features when depressed. Atypical symptoms are also common in people who merit the qualifier "with seasonal pattern" (Seasonal Affective Disorder, SAD in nontechnical terms). Patient II is thus at greatest increased risk for a seasonal pattern or for manic episodes. It would be unusual for the older patients to have first manic episodes so late in life (though they would be at risk if they had had previous ones). Patient VI has a chronic, low-grade, persistent illness, rather than an episodic one.

Patient III has an **adjustment disorder with depressed mood**. There is an identifiable precipitant to his symptoms, he does not have a full-blown depressive syndrome, and his symptoms have not lasted more than six months.

Patient IV has a **major depressive episode with melancholic features**, specifically early morning awakening, anhedonia, diurnal variation with mornings worse, suicidal ideation, and guilt. Her mood differs from normal grief.

Middle aged and older women are unduly prone to autoimmune disease, including thyroiditis. Hypothyroidism is high in the medical differential diagnosis of someone with either atypical or melancholic depression, especially if the person also has hypercholesterolemia. The high cholesterol does not cause the mood symptoms, but may be a marker for the thyroid dysfunction. LH/FSH are tests for documentation of menopause. They would undoubtedly be elevated in patient IV, but of no diagnostic value. Whether recent menopause may precipitate depression in vulnerable women is a matter of some debate. The majority of perimenopausal women, however, experience only mild, transient mood symptoms. Well-established menopause is not an adequate cause for a major depressive episode. Major depression with melancholia is associated with abnormal cortisol metabolism in roughly 50% of cases, but a single value would be uninterpretable. A dexamethasone- suppression test would be required to uncover the abnormality.

Patient **V** illustrates **dysthymic disorder**, a state of persistent mood symptoms more days than not, some vegetative symptoms but not a full depressive syndrome, and negative views of self and the future.

Patient **VI** illustrates **major depression with mood congruent psychotic features** (accusatory hallucinations and delusions of poverty). The patient does not have a history of psychotic symptoms in the absence of depressed mood. Thus, she is not schizoaffective, depressed, the only other diagnosis on the list that might merit consideration.

Items 302-309

Choose the **BEST** response.

302.   Among depressed patients, more thorough medical evaluation is required in those

    (A)   over fifty experiencing a first episode
    (B)   who lack a family history of depression
    (C)   who also have somatic complaints pointing to possible medical diagnoses
    (D)   A and C only
    (E)   A, B, and C

303.   Major depression and its subtypes may occur in all the following medical conditions **EXCEPT**:

    (A)   viral infections (mononucleosis, viral hepatitis, HIV and related infections)
    (B)   regular sedative (benzodiazepine or barbiturate) use
    (C)   valvular heart disease, including mitral valve prolapse
    (D)   endocrine imbalances especially hypo/hyperthyroidism; hyper/hypoadrenalism
    (E)   heavy metal poisoning

140

304. Depressed patients may also have symptoms suggesting dementia and dementing patients may become depressed. The dementia syndrome of depression (formerly pseudodementia) differs from depression occurring as part of a dementing illness in

   (A) leading to scores in the normal range on the Mini-Mental State Examination (MMSE)
   (B) the complete absence of signs of cortical atrophy on CT scan
   (C) partial reversibility with antidepressant treatment
   (D) the tendency of depressed patients to minimize their cognitive complaints, compared to mental status findings
   (E) All of the above

305. Identify the other **TRUE** statement(s) comparing primary dementia/dementia syndrome of depression.

   (A) Patients with the dementia syndrome of depression more typically have a history of previous episodes of depression.
   (B) Patients with primary dementia try harder to answer questions; patients with the dementia syndrome of depression give more "don't know" answers.
   (C) Primary dementia has a more insidious onset.
   (D) If diurnal variation is present, depressed patients will typically feel worse in the morning; demented patients worsen in the evenings.
   (E) All of the above

306. Although depression may occur without any physical findings, all the following have been found in depression and may be markers of the illness **EXCEPT**:

   (A) decreased REM latency and reduced stage 3 and 4 sleep on sleep EEG
   (B) early cortisol escape from dexamethasone suppression
   (C) loss of normal diurnal cycles of cortisol secretion with tonically high cortisol output
   (D) increased TSH response to the infusion of TRH
   (E) decreased levels of the 5-HT metabolite 5-HIAA in the cerebrospinal fluid

307. While the research tests above occasionally help confirm a clinical diagnosis of depression, screening for these abnormalities is not part of a standard work-up for depression because the tests

   (A) have inadequate sensitivity or specificity
   (B) are too expensive
   (C) are too invasive
   (D) A and C only
   (E) A, B, and C

308. All the following support the role of reduced serotonin neurotransmission in the pathophysiology of some depressions **EXCEPT**:

(A) efficacy of bupropion in treating depression
(B) reduction of central and peripheral (platelet) 5-HT reuptake sites in untreated, depressed patients
(C) blunting of serum prolactin response to serotonin in depression
(D) low levels of 5-HIAA in the CSF of up to 40% of depressed patients
(E) efficacy of fluoxetine and related drugs in the treatment of depression

309. The finding of low 5-HIAA in the CSF is also associated with

(A) completed suicide
(B) dementia-like symptoms
(C) impulsive aggression
(D) A and C only
(E) A, B, and C

ANSWERS AND TUTORIAL ON ITEMS 302-309

The answers are: **302-D; 303-C; 304-C; 305-E; 306-D; 307-E; 308-A; 309-D**. As indicated by its mix of cognitive and physical symptoms, depression is a psychobiological state. This implies both that depression may occur in the context of systemic medical illnesses and also that certain physical or laboratory abnormalities may occur.

The **onset of depression**, like the onset of serious medical illness, rises steadily with age. Even when depression is the chief complaint and a full depressive syndrome is present, careful review of systems at any age may uncover symptoms such as sore throat (viral illness), changes in hair or skin or menstrual function (endocrine disorders), snoring (sleep apnea), or joint pain and swelling (autoimmune disease) suggestive of medical conditions known to present with depression. Thus, advancing age (especially at first onset) or particular physical symptoms require intensified medical screening. Although genetic studies show that depression may run in families, this finding is too variable to help the clinician decide if depression in a given patient is idiopathic (presumed an expression of genetic factors) or occurring secondary to medical illness.

Essentially any **systemic condition** (viremia, toxins, metabolic imbalances, autoimmune disease) can cause mental status changes, including depression. Isolated organ dysfunction is much less likely to be a contributory cause. When echocardiography first made it possible to diagnose mitral valve prolapse reliably, some investigators thought this finding might relate to panic disorder (not depression). The relationship turned out to be artifactual. Panic attacks and mitral valve prolapse are both most common in women between the ages of 20 and 40, hence their statistical association.

The **dementia syndrome of depression** connotes the memory loss, decreased concentration, and slowed thinking seen in depressed patients. Differentiating this from **primary dementia** can be difficult, since dementia may entail symptoms that overlap with depression, including apathy, disrupted sleep, changes in appetite, irritability, and easy tearfulness. Most of the points differentiating the two diagnoses are matters of degree. Thus, the MMSE scores of depressed patients with cognitive symptoms fall between those of normal (>25) and demented (<15) patients. Patients with primary dementing illness are typically unaware of the extent of their deficits. Patients with depression are hypersensitive to signs of impairment and will exaggerate (not minimize) their complaints, leading to better than expected performance on the mental status examination. Cortical atrophy on CT scans is not a reliable differentiating finding-- patients with considerable signs of atrophy may have normal mentation and demented patients may show no anatomical atrophy, especially in the early stages of their illness. Moreover, symptoms of dementia occur more in older depressed patients than younger ones, and radiographic signs of atrophy rise with age. The main differentiating point is therefore the reversibility of the dementia symptoms with antidepressant treatment. This reversal need not be complete; patients who seem demented when depressed often have persistent, age appropriate cognitive loss when the depression is treated.

Primary dementia differs further from the dementia syndrome of depression in being of more insidious onset. Demented patients are less likely to give "don't know" answers to test questions and are less likely to have a previous history of depressive episodes. The diurnal patterns of the two conditions helps to differentiate them: demented patients worsen in the evening ("sundowning"); depressed patients (especially melancholic subtype) feel worst on awakening and may improve somewhat as the day goes on.

Item 306 lists the physical markers of depression found in research studies; TSH response to TRH infusion may be **blunted** in depressed patients, making (D) the only incorrect answer. The problem with the endocrine tests is that they lack both sensitivity (up to 50% false negatives) and specificity (similar endocrine abnormalities may be found, though at lower rates, in related psychiatric conditions). Endocrine tests are also relatively invasive--the TRH stimulation test requires an indwelling IV for several hours and the dexamethasone-suppression test requires the patient to take dexamethasone and have at least one if not several venipunctures. Though sensitive and specific enough for clinical use, sleep EEGs are expensive and cumbersome. A systematic, careful interview is still the best screening test for depression. A clinical physical examination and routine lab work will rule out the most common associated medical conditions. Other investigations, though of interest in elucidating the pathophysiology of depression, are reserved for atypical cases and for the evaluation of people who do not respond as expected to adequate treatment.

All the answers in Item 308 except A support the role of **serotonin in the etiology of depression**. **Bupropion** is the only antidepressant with no known effect on serotonergic function. Its efficacy in depression suggests that other neurotransmitters besides serotonin are also likely to be involved.

The finding of low levels of the serotonin metabolite **5-HIAA** in CSF is not specific to depression. Serotonin tends to inhibit aggression in normal animals and in man. Decreased 5-HIAA (a marker of decreased serotonin turnover) may be associated with increased aggression of any type (self- or other-directed) in a variety of psychiatric conditions and in those without definable mental illness. Serotonin function has either not been studied or not found to be particularly associated with cognitive impairment, so in Item 309 answer B is incorrect.

Items 310-316

The following set of items pertains to bipolar disorder. Choose the **BEST** response.

310. All the following are among the criteria for a manic episode **EXCEPT**:

   (A)   at least a week of euphoric, expansive, or irritable mood
   (B)   narrowing of attention to the point of preoccupation
   (C)   overtalkativeness
   (D)   decreased need for sleep
   (E)   excessive involvement in pleasurable activities (sex, spending) despite a high potential for painful consequences

311. A manic episode differs from a hypomanic episode

   (A)   in lasting longer (at least one week compared to four days)
   (B)   in causing marked functional impairment or leading to hospitalization
   (C)   in sometimes having psychotic features
   (D)   A and C only
   (E)   A, B, and C

312. Patients with bipolar II disorder

   (A)   experience recurrent depressions
   (B)   experience hypomanic episodes
   (C)   differ from patients with cyclothymic disorder in having full-blown depressive episodes
   (D)   A and C only
   (E)   A, B, and C

313. Rapid cycling

(A) is defined as a person having four episodes of depression, mania, hypomania or a mixed state in a year
(B) is more common in men than women
(C) may be induced by the use of antidepressants
(D) A and C only
(E) A, B, and C

314. The term schizoaffective disorder, most recent episode manic, connotes someone

(A) who simultaneously meets criteria for a schizophrenic disorder and a manic episode
(B) with mood incongruent psychotic features while manic
(C) with a history of both a recent manic episode and of psychotic symptoms occurring when he/she is not in either a manic or depressive episode
(D) with schizophrenia who has a family history of bipolar disorder
(E) with bipolar disorder who has a family history of schizophrenia

315. All the following are **TRUE** statements **EXCEPT**:

(A) First degree relatives with bipolar disorder are more common in the families of bipolar patients than in the families of normal controls.
(B) Unipolar and bipolar disorders are equally common in the first degree relatives of unipolar depressed patients.
(C) Bipolar patients have excess numbers of first degree relatives with both bipolar disorder and unipolar disorders.
(D) Schizophrenia is no more common in the families of bipolar patients than in the families of normal controls.
(E) Genetic factors probably play a greater role in bipolar disorders than in unipolar ones.

316. The medical differential diagnosis of a manic or hypomanic episode includes

(A) hyperthyroidism
(B) cocaine or amphetamine abuse
(C) Cushing's disease (hypercortisolemia)
(D) All of the above
(E) None of the above

ANSWERS AND TUTORIAL ON ITEMS 310-316

The answers are: **310-B; 311-E; 312-E; 313-D; 314-C; 315-B; 316-D**. Since antiquity, physicians have recognized that some patients experience both depressive episodes and episodes of excitement, increased energy, decreased need for sleep, and impulsivity. Kraepelin is credited with describing this pattern in modern terms and in noting that, in contrast to schizophrenia, patients with extreme mood swings do not typically follow a deteriorating course.

The **manic state**, by definition, includes both core mood symptoms--euphoria, irritability, or expansiveness--and neurovegetative changes: decreased need for sleep, increased energy, hypertalkativeness, changes in eating (weight loss or weight gain), and increased impulsivity, often leading to increased sexual activity or increased spending. Manic patients are typically distractible. Intensification of concentration is, therefore, not a defining symptom.

Elevated moods are subclassified as **manic**, with or without psychotic features, and **hypomanic**. The presence of mood congruent psychotic features during a manic episode seems to be a marker of severity, and does not worsen the prognosis for recovery. Hypomanic states, which were only precisely defined in DSM-IV, are milder and briefer than mania. They are, by definition, nonpsychotic and do not impair function, although they must, again by definition, represent a clear, recognizable change from baseline.

DSM-IV recognizes at least three different forms of alternating mood disorder: **bipolar or bipolar I**; **bipolar II**; and **cyclothymic disorder**. Bipolar I differs from bipolar II in having full-blown manic, rather than hypomanic episodes. Cyclothymic disorder differs from both in that neither the depressed nor the elevated phases meet full criteria for manic or major depressive episode. The rapid cycling qualifier, connoting four or more discreet mood episodes in a year, represents another recognized subtype. Rapid cycling is more common in women than in men. It may be induced by antidepressant treatment and may be more refractory to treatment with lithium than other forms of bipolar disorder.

Genetics seem to play a greater role in bipolar than unipolar depressive disorders. Bipolar patients have increased rates of both unipolar and bipolar depression in their relatives; unipolar patients, by contrast, tend to have unipolar but not bipolar relatives. This finding partly reflects that unipolar depression is 10 times more common than bipolar disorder and also more heterogeneous; any population of unipolar patients will include a much higher percentage of sporadic (nongenetic) cases, so that the number of patients with bipolar relatives will be small relative to the total. It is noteworthy that mood disorders are not associated with higher familial risk for other severe mental illnesses like schizophrenia.

Like depression, mania can be secondary to a systemic medical illness or condition. Stimulant intoxication, hyperthyroidism, and hypercortisolism are all recognized causes of manic syndromes. Almost any process affecting the CNS can cause mania, which has been reported from HIV and related infections, multiple sclerosis, uremia, and syphilis. However, depression or delirium are more common than mania as sequelae of severe medical illness.

Items 317-333

The following items pertain to the treatment of mood disorders.

Items 317-326

Match the drugs in the answers below with the **MOST** appropriate descriptive phrase in the items. Answers may be used once, more than once, or not at all.

(A) Fluoxetine, paroxetine, sertraline
(B) Amitriptyline, imipramine
(C) Nortriptyline, desipramine
(D) Bupropion
(E) Nefazodone
(F) Trazodone
(G) Tranylcypromine; phenelzine
(H) Lithium, valproic acid, carbamazepine
(I) Venlafaxine
(J) Clomipramine

317. Antidepressants that inhibit monoamine oxidase, raising levels of norepinephrine and serotonin by preventing their catabolism.

318. Only dopaminergic antidepressant; does not affect serotonin or norepinephrine levels.

319. Examples of earliest antidepressants; block the reuptake of norepinephrine and serotonin.

320. Associated, albeit rarely, with priapism in men; very sedating; first antidepressant that was safe in overdose.

321. New antidepressant thought to be useful in patients who do not respond to more selective drugs (e.g., serotonin-specific reuptake inhibitors); only antidepressant typically associated with hypertension.

322. Highly anticholinergic and antihistaminic antidepressants, often producing unacceptable side-effects; lethal in overdose.

323. Typically lowers blood pressure but may cause dangerous, even lethal hypertension in combination with foods containing tyramine; lethally interacts with meperidine or serotonergic drugs.

324. Active metabolite of older antidepressants with fewer side-effects; still potentially lethal in overdose.

325. Effective treatment for mania and sometimes effective for the depressed phase of bipolar illness.

Choose the **BEST** response.

326. The choice of antidepressant medication for a given patient is governed by

 (A)   symptom pattern and severity
 (B)   past personal or family member's response to a given drug
 (C)   nature of coexisting medical problems
 (D)   A and C only
 (E)   A, B, and C

Items 327-330

Match the pattern of toxicity described in the answers below with the **MOST** appropriate involved neurotransmitter in the items. Answers may be used once, more than once, or not at all

 (A)   Diarrhea, fever, myoclonus, delirium, hypertension, sweating
 (B)   Constipation, dry mouth, blurred vision, urinary retention, dilated pupils, dry skin, increased temperature, delirium, heart block, arrhythmias, seizures
 (C)   Severe hypertension, headache, stroke
 (D)   Fever, elevated WBC, fluctuations in blood pressure, tachypnea, sweating, elevated creatinine phosphokinase (CPK)

327. Serotonin

328. Acetylcholine

329. Dopamine

330. Tyramine

Choose the **BEST** response.

331. "Second generation" antidepressants (nontricyclic, non-MAO inhibiting) are preferable to older agents because

  (A) They have a shorter response latency (immediate as opposed to delayed symptom relief).
  (B) They are more effective.
  (C) They are safer and better tolerated.
  (D) All of the above
  (E) None of the above

332. A depression that does not respond to a given medication is considered refractory. In treating a refractory depression, the clinician

  (A) Should ensure adequate dosing by raising the dose to the highest tolerable level guided, when possible, by serum drug levels .
  (B) Should discontinue medication and try psychotherapy alone.
  (C) Should switch to a different class of antidepressant.
  (D) A and C only
  (E) A, B, and C

333. Other treatments for refractory depression include

  (A) augmentation of antidepressant with lithium
  (B) electroconvulsive therapy
  (C) augmentation with thyroid hormone, especially T_3
  (D) A and C only
  (E) A, B, and C

ANSWERS AND TUTORIAL ON ITEMS 317-333

The answers are: **317-G; 318-D; 319-B; 320-F; 321-I; 322-B; 323-G; 324-C; 325-H; 326-E; 327-A; 328-B; 329-D; 330-C; 331-C; 332-D; 333-E**. Current pharmacologic treatments for depression include three distinct classes of antidepressant drugs and a handful of unique or novel agents. The three classes are the **cyclic antidepressants** (TCAs or CyADs), **monoamine oxidase**

inhibitors (MAOIs), and **serotonin-specific reuptake inhibitors** (SSRIs). CyADs are subdivided into the tertiary amine tricyclics (amitriptyline, imipramine, doxepin, clomipramine, trimipramine), secondary amine metabolites (nortriptyline, protriptyline, desipramine), and tetracyclics (amoxapine, maprotiline). MAOIs include phenelzine, tranylcypromine, and isocarboxazid. Fluoxetine, paroxetine, fluvoxamine, sertraline, and mirtazapine comprise the SSRIs.

Drugs and drug classes vary mainly in pharmacokinetics, side-effects, and lethality in overdose. All increase synaptic levels of monamine neurotransmitters, by blocking reuptake (CyAD, SSRIs), inhibiting catabolism (MAOIs), or direct stimulation (trazodone, nefazodone). Flooding the synapse precipitates side-effects, which may be immediate. Antidepressant effects correlate in time with the neuronal reaction to persistently increased levels of neurotransmitters, specifically downregulation of postsynaptic and feedback receptors, especially β-adrenergic receptors. β-adrenergic receptor downregulation occurs with all the currently available drugs, including the SSRIs. For this reason, although antidepressants differ meaningfully in terms of side-effects and toxicity, all have roughly similar response latency (time to remission) and equal efficacy.

Information about pharmacokinetics, side-effects, and toxicity can be organized according to class of drug--the novel agents must be learned separately. CyADs all have anticholinergic and antihistaminic side-effects, especially sedation, orthostatic hypotension, dry mouth, constipation, urinary retention, sexual dysfunction, and weight gain. Abrupt discontinuation may produce cholinergic rebound effects--nausea, vomiting, diarrhea, and sleeplessness. Immediate increase in synaptic norepinephrine probably explains why these drugs (especially imipramine and desipramine) produce anxiety (which they may later relieve, due to downregulation).

Nortriptyline, desipramine, and protriptyline are all active, secondary amine metabolites of tricyclics with similar, but significantly milder, side-effects. Clomipramine is chlorinated imipramine (not a metabolite) with unique efficacy for obsessive-compulsive symptoms but also very severe anticholinergic and antihistaminic side-effects. Amoxapine has antidopaminergic effects and is associated with the risk of extrapyramidal side-effects and tardive dyskinesia.

MAOIs have relatively few anticholinergic side-effects, though they may cause orthostatic hypotension (by blockade of α-adrenergic receptors), weight gain, agitation and impotence/anorgasmia.

The SSRIs have become the drugs of first choice in the treatment of depression largely because of their milder side-effects and the lack of significant toxicity, even in overdose. Side-effects include agitation/sleeplessness (occasionally sedation), nausea/vomiting or milder loss of appetite and weight, sexual dysfunction, and headache. These drugs do not affect blood pressure or cardiac conduction.

Among the novel agents, the mechanism of action of bupropion appears to be blockade of dopamine receptors. This drug has mild side-effects--sleeplessness, weight loss--and shares with nefazodone the advantage of not causing sexual dysfunction. Its main toxicity is the potential to cause seizures in high doses, requiring divided doses during the day.

Trazodone and nefazodone, which are both serotonin reuptake blockers and serotonin agonists, differ more than one would expect, given their fundamental similarities. Trazodone is very sedating and may be given adjunctively (in low doses) to improve sleep in depressed patients on nonsedating drugs like bupropion or the SSRIs. Trazodone lacks anticholinergic and

150

antihistaminic effects on blood pressure and the heart and was the first antidepressant that was safe in overdose. It's unique liability is the possibility of causing priapism--a fixed, painful erection in men that may require surgery and lead to permanent sexual dysfunction. This complication occurs rarely, and men who have sexual dysfunction with other antidepressants may tolerate trazodone better. Nefazodone seems to have less of trazodone's sedating properties and causes no sexual dysfunction, although it may cause nausea. It competes with terfenadine and astemizole for metabolism by a cytochrome P_{450} enzyme and may interact lethally (via cardiac arrhythmia--*torsade de pointes*) with these drugs.

Venlafaxine blocks the reuptake of both norepinephrine and serotonin but lacks the anticholinergic properties of the tricyclics. It may cause nausea, somnolence or insomnia, and is the only antidepressant that may cause hypertension in therapeutic doses.

The mood stabilizers (lithium and the anticonvulsants carbamazepine and valproic acid) are included with this review of antidepressants because they often prevent and occasionally relieve depression in patients who are bipolar. Lithium, in addition, has been used to augment the effects of tricyclics and MAOIs, sometimes converting drug-refractory patients to drug-responders.

As noted above, some antidepressants have unique or idiosyncratic drug interactions and toxicities as well as side-effects. Some patterns of toxicity reflect syndromes related to particular neurotransmitters: anticholinergic delirium, the serotonin syndrome, neuroleptic malignant syndrome (a dopaminergic toxicity relevant to antipsychotics, see Chapter VI), and the effects of tyramine acting as a false transmitter. Anticholinergic toxicity (CyADs) includes delayed cardiac conduction, precipitation of acute glaucoma, and delirium, with dilated pupils, hot dry skin, constipation, and urinary retention. The "serotonin syndrome"--diarrhea, fever, myoclonus, confusion, hypertension, and diaphoresis--occurs mainly when MAOIs are combined with serotonergic drugs. Switching patients from SSRIs or MAOIs to the alternate drug requires prolonged washout periods; combinations of these drugs should never be given.

MAO catabolizes **tyramine**, a pressor amine found in a variety of fermented foods including wine, most cheeses, and some legumes. When MAO is inhibited, patients who ingest tyramine-containing foods may experience severe, paroxysmal hypertension, leading to stroke or death. A similar reaction may also occur when patients ingest sympathomimetic drugs, including ephedrine in over-the-counter cold preparations. MAOIs also interact lethally with the narcotic meperidine by an unknown mechanism.

Dopamine, or dopamine blockade, is involved in the pathophysiology of the neuroleptic malignant syndrome (fever, delirium, rigidity, tachypnea, elevated CPK and WBCs) Amoxapine is the only antidepressant with dopamine blocking properties.

Skillful clinical use of antidepressants involves trying to capitalize on their side-effects for therapeutic benefit, awareness of toxicity and particular advantages or liabilities, and protocols for handling the problem of patients' nonresponse to a given agent. The first principle is "give enough for long enough." All antidepressant effects are dose dependent and all available drugs have significant response latency (marketing claims to the contrary notwithstanding). While immediate improvement may occur, sustained improvement may be delayed for three to six weeks after starting treatment.

The most common prescribing error is underdosing or giving up too soon. Tricyclic effects have been correlated with blood levels, which can be measured clinically. With all other drugs, finding the appropriate or adequate dose requires trial and error. Patients' response to a three week trial of a standard "threshold" dose is determined first. Nonresponsive patients should then have their dose raised to a maximum level based on tolerance for side-effects. Treatment must continue another three weeks before the physician can conclude that a given drug is ineffective.

Various patterns of symptoms appear to respond to certain antidepressants more than others. Patterns of side-effects help predict which drug may work best--patients with disrupted sleep do better with sedating drugs, patients who have lost weight will have greater tolerance for drugs that produce weight gain, and so on. More systematic studies have shown that patients with atypical features (hypersomnia, retardation, weight gain) respond better to MAOIs and possibly SSRIs than to tricyclics; melancholic features respond preferentially to tricyclics and possibly venlafaxine.

Because the guidelines for choosing antidepressants are so empirical, the best predictor of patients' response is their own past personal history with various classes of drugs. In a first episode, the history of family members' medication responses or nonresponses may help. The existence of concurrent medical problems also affects the choice of antidepressant. Elderly patients, in particular, may have low tolerance for drugs with anticholinergic side-effects and also for drugs commonly involved in drug-drug interactions.

When patients do not respond to a sustained trial of an antidepressant at an adequate dose, it is an error to conclude they are completely drug-refractory and should be treated with psychotherapy alone. Augmentation of the primary drug with lithium or L-triiodothyronine (T_3) may convert a nonresponder into a responder. Changing from one class of antidepressant to another may also be effective. Changes from an MAOI to a TCA or SSRI require a two week washout to avoid severe toxic interactions. Finally, electroconvulsive therapy remains the most effective treatment for depression and may induce remission in patients who have failed to respond to trials of various drugs and combinations.

Choose the **BEST** response.

334. Which of the following subtypes specifically indicates the need for somatic treatment?

    (A)   depression with psychotic features
    (B)   depression with melancholic features
    (C)   depressed phase of bipolar disorder
    (D)   A and C only
    (E)   A, B, and C

335. Psychopharmacologic treatment is contraindicated in

    (A)   dysthymic disorder
    (B)   adjustment disorder with depressed mood
    (C)   depression in patients with personality disorders
    (D)   All of the above
    (E)   None of the above

336. Both brief interpersonal therapy and brief cognitive therapy

    (A)   are as effective as antidepressants for unqualified, mild to moderate depression
    (B)   are compatible with concurrent use of antidepressants or other somatic treatment
    (C)   have demonstrated some prophylactic effects, delaying the time to recurrence or relapse, especially if given in a maintenance format
    (D)   A and C only
    (E)   A, B, and C

337. Psychotherapy for depression

    (A)   may produce continuing improvement months after treatment ends
    (B)   may equal medication in relief of mild to moderate vegetative symptoms
    (C)   exceeds medication treatment in improving social functioning
    (D)   A and C only
    (E)   A, B, and C

ANSWERS AND TUTORIAL ON ITEMS 334-337

The answers are: **334-E; 335-E; 336-E; 337-E. Depression** is a psychobiological state. All clinically significant mood disorders, by definition, involve bodily symptoms (vegetative changes and the core abnormal mood), recognizably distorted patterns of thought (negative view of self and the future), and disruptions in social relations (losses, unsatisfying or conflicted attachments, loneliness). Different modalities of treatment address each aspect. In mild to moderate unipolar depression, **psychotherapy** that focuses on either the cognitive or interpersonal dimensions may bring about remission of all symptoms over time, including the vegetative symptoms. In melancholic, psychotic or bipolar depression, antidepressant or mood-stabilizing **medication** is necessary. Psychotherapy alone is usually ineffective.

In other forms of depression, the decision to use or not use medication is always provisional. Although dysthymic or personality disordered patients may have few vegetative symptoms, some respond surprisingly well to antidepressants. Adjustment disorders, though by definition understandable reactions to disruptive events, still sometimes resolve more quickly with pharmacologic treatment for depressive (or anxiety) symptoms. The decision whether or not to use medication, then, is based not on diagnosis, but on the presence or absence of symptoms that may respond to it. Another element of the decision is patients' response or nonresponse to other forms of treatment.

Despite some concerns that giving antidepressants might diminish patients' motivation to participate in psychotherapy, most clinicians view the combination as synergistic. Cognitive distortions in depression sometimes improve on medication alone and sometimes with psychotherapy alone. If psychotherapy is not part of the treatment, improvement in interpersonal relations either does not occur or occurs after much delay. Medication does not by itself teach patients how to recognize depressive patterns of thought or relationships or provide ways of avoiding them. Drugs act only while taken. Psychotherapy, by contrast, produces continuing improvement after the end of treatment, as patients put their insights into practice. Psychotherapy in some studies is prophylactic, delaying and perhaps preventing the onset of the next episode.

Items 338-344

Choose the **BEST** response.

338. Electroconvulsive therapy (ECT) is the **BEST** treatment for

    (A)   chronic schizophrenia, paranoid type
    (B)   phencyclidine intoxication
    (C)   mood disorder secondary to cocaine dependence
    (D)   melancholic depression
    (E)   bipolar disorder

339. The person who statistically will respond **BEST** to ECT is

    (A)   an 18-year-old male with a first psychotic break
    (B)   an 82-year-old woman with psychotic depression and multiple medical problems
    (C)   a 34-year-old male in the depressive phase of bipolar disorder
    (D)   a 15-year-old girl with adjustment disorder with depressed mood
    (E)   a 50-year-old alcoholic man who is depressed and suicidal

340. All of the following are **RELATIVE** contraindications to ECT **EXCEPT**:

    (A)   recent myocardial infarction (within 6 weeks)
    (B)   intracranial mass
    (C)   pregnancy
    (D)   subarachnoid hemorrhage
    (E)   pacemaker

341. Which of the following have been postulated as probable reasons for the efficacy of ECT?

    (A)   the seizure releases endogenous opiates which may ameliorate depressed mood
    (B)   induction of seizure causes massive release of catecholamines into synapses, mimicking the effect of antidepressant medications
    (C)   repeated seizures induce down regulation of postsynaptic β-adrenergic receptors
    (D)   A and C only
    (E)   A, B, and C

342. Which of the following correlates **MOST** closely with the therapeutic effect of ECT?

   (A)   intensity of current delivered
   (B)   method of seizure induction
   (C)   induction of generalized tonic-clonic seizure
   (D)   electrical qualities of a particular ECT machine
   (E)   seizure that is detected by EEG and not by muscular contractions

343. Which of the following constitutes an **ABSOLUTE** contraindication for ECT?

   (A)   recent cerebrovascular accident
   (B)   meningioma
   (C)   severe hypertension
   (D)   recent myocardial infarction
   (E)   None of the above

344. Bradycardia during ECT is thought to be due to

   (A)   sympathetic discharge that follows the seizure
   (B)   parasympathetic discharge that follows stimulus delivery
   (C)   sympathetic discharge that follows stimulus delivery
   (D)   A and C only
   (E)   None of the above

ANSWERS AND TUTORIAL ON ITEMS 338-344

The answers are: **338-D; 339-B; 340-C; 341-E; 342-C; 343-E; 344-B. Electroconvulsive therapy** (ECT) is a treatment modality that has been gravely under-utilized due, in part, to lack of clear knowledge of how it works and the negative image created by the media for the general public. In fact, ECT is highly effective, safe and, at times, a life-saving procedure for the treatment of severe depression. The effective element of the treatment is the seizure itself, not the method of induction or monitoring. While a number of conditions including bipolar disorder and acute psychotic states can respond to ECT, melancholic depression in the elderly, especially with psychotic features, is the condition for which ECT is the treatment of choice.

   While ECT can benefit a variety of patients, statistical predictors of good outcome identify the population most likely to respond. Among these are advanced age, melancholic depression especially with psychotic features, previous history of good response to ECT, family history of good response to ECT, and absence of severe personality disorder. If schizophrenia is present, predictors of favorable ECT response include: the acute onset of symptoms, prominence of mood symptoms, and the presence of positive symptoms of psychosis (delusions, hallucinations, agitation, disorganized behavior).

Although ECT is an extremely safe procedure with the risks of side-effects being less than that of standard pharmacological treatments, some relative contraindications exist. They mostly relate to the risk of anaesthesia and the physiological effects of a seizure. Since a seizure transiently increases intracranial pressure (ICP), the conditions that also increase ICP (intracranial mass, intracranial hemorrhage) constitute relative contraindications. This means that ECT can be done, but with extra precautions, including immediately available resuscitation. Additionally, seizures cause a systemic release of catecholamines, with resultant increases in blood pressure and heart rate. Patients who are hypertensive or are recovering from myocardial infarction are, thus, at a greater risk of untoward effects.

The most common untoward effects of ECT are postictal confusion including retrograde amnesia and, less frequently, arrhythmias including ventricular tachycardia and ventricular fibrillation. The irregularities of heart beat are due to autonomic hyperactivity. Administration of the electrical stimulus produces a profound parasympathetic outflow which slows the heart rate early in the procedure. The seizure itself causes a sympathetic outflow with concomitant increase in heart rate, especially during the later phase of the procedure and in the immediate recovery period.

Items 345-350

Match the drug in the answers below with the **BEST** descriptive phrase in the items. Answers may be used once, more than once, or not at all.

   (A) Phenobarbital
   (B) Succinylcholine
   (C) Ethambutol
   (D) Methohexital
   (E) Propaphol
   (F) Glycopyrrolate
   (G) Phenytoin
   (H) Diphenhydramine
   (I) Diazepam
   (J) Tubocurarine

345. Barbiturate anaesthetic most commonly used during electroconvulsive therapy (ECT).

346. The agent which is used to abort status epilepticus and to stop prolonged seizures during ECT.

347. An agent used prior to ECT to decrease secretions and prevent the emergence of early bradyarrhythmias.

348. Short-acting paralytic agent which is employed during ECT to minimize muscular contractions and prevent spinal fractures.

349. Congenital absence of acetylcholinesterase may prolong resumption of spontaneous respiration after using this agent.

350. While this anaesthetic agent has gained popularity as an agent of choice for short surgical procedures, its use in ECT is limited because of the drug's effects on seizure threshold and duration.

ANSWERS AND TUTORIAL ON ITEMS 345-350

The answers are: **345-D; 346-I; 347-F; 348-B; 349-B; 350-E. Methohexital** (D) is an ultra short-acting barbiturate. It is used in a number of procedures which are brief and do not require deep anaesthesia. Its particular utility in ECT reflects methohexital's minimal effect on seizure threshold. Other barbiturates and propaphol tend to increase the seizure threshold and shorten the duration of convulsions. Additionally, methohexital is not associated with confusion upon reversal of anaesthesia. It is particularly helpful in ECT, which already produces a confused state.

While **status epilepticus** is an extremely rare complication of ECT, a seizure in excess of two minutes is not desirable. It increases the chances of hypoxia, postictal confusion and a general hypometabolic state. As is true with idiopathic epilepsy, the drug used intravenously to abort a prolonged seizure is **diazepam** (I). It is extremely fast acting, yet has a half- life of four to six hours. Its CNS activity is almost immediate upon intravenous administration. Phenytoin (G) requires a loading procedure, CNS accumulation, and **slow** intravenous administration for effectiveness as an anticonvulsant. While quite useful in long-term control of seizures, the immediate efficacy of phenytoin is questionable.

Glycopyrrolate is a relatively short-acting ($t_{1/2}$ = 2-4 hours) anticholinergic agent. It is frequently administered just prior to induction of anaesthesia. As any anticholinergic agent, it blocks parasympathetic outflow to respiratory, cardiac, and digestive organs. As such, it decreases respiratory secretions and saliva, making aspiration less likely. It also prevents vagal slowing of the heart, thus preventing early bradyarrhythmias.

Succinylcholine (B) is an ultrashort-acting depolarizing agent that works at the motor end-plate, preventing muscle contraction. Its use made ECT a much safer procedure by preventing spinal fractures, which occasionally would occur due to strong muscular contractions. **Tubocurarine** (J), while also paralytic, tends to be long-acting and is not metabolized by the end of ECT. This leaves the patient awake, yet paralyzed. Because of its long duration of action and the need for intubation, the use of tubocurarine is limited in ECT.

Acetylcholine, a neurotransmitter responsible for the chain of events resulting in muscle contraction, is broken down by the enzyme acetylcholinesterase. The same enzyme breaks down succinylcholine. In individuals with congenital deficiency of this enzyme, succinylcholine is broken down at a slower rate, thus prolonging muscle paralysis. Failure to resume spontaneous breathing after ECT may result from an inborn deficiency of acetylcholinesterase which was unknown prior to the procedure.

Propaphol (E), as was mentioned earlier, is a new ultrashort-acting nonbarbiturate anaesthetic. It is used widely in brief outpatient procedures not requiring deep anesthesia. It reverses spontaneously upon discontinuation of intravenous drip. Moreover, it causes little nausea, confusion or sedation, making it, in principle, an ideal anaesthetic agent for ECT. However, it has been known to raise the seizure threshold and shorten the duration of seizures, thus requiring higher doses of electricity to induce a therapeutic seizure. Higher electrical doses lead to increased delirium and memory loss, making propaphol not a useful agent in this procedure.

Items 351-358

Matching

     (A)   Unilateral nondominant ECT
     (B)   Bilateral ECT
     (C)   Both
     (D)   Neither

351.   More effective method to induce electrical seizures.

352.   Used for the treatment of severe recurrent major depression in the elderly especially when complicated by the presence of psychosis.

353.   Is more effective than an average antidepressant medication for the treatment of depression.

354.   Is used in treatment of refractory cases.

355.   Has been know to induce a manic state.

356.   Is associated with **greater** postictal confusion, memory loss and agitation.

357.   Requires informed consent.

358.   Is the treatment of choice for diffuse identity disorder.

ANSWERS AND TUTORIAL ON ITEMS 351-358

The answers are: **351-B; 352-C; 353-C; 354-B; 355-C; 356-B; 357-C; 358-D**. There are a number of differences between **bilateral** and **unilateral ECT** both in terms of treatment efficacy and side-effect profile. Bilateral stimulus placement enhances the likelihood of induction of a generalized tonic-clonic seizure. As such, it is a more effective method than unilateral stimulus placement for seizure induction and is used in treatment-resistant cases. Clinically, the only differences in indications for bilateral ECT vs. unilateral ECT are:

1) treatment refractoriness after unilateral ECT
2) inability to induce seizure with unilateral stimulation
3) history of better past response to bilateral ECT

When compared to standard antidepressant therapy for major depression, both unilateral and bilateral ECT boast greater effectiveness, with bilateral ECT being more effective than unilateral. Both treatment modalities have been known to precipitate mania in bipolar depressed patients, with bilateral ECT slightly leading in incidence. While bilateral ECT is more efficacious, it is also associated with greater side-effects. It increases the likelihood of confusion, delirium and memory loss. Informed consent is required for both procedures, as it is for initiation of pharmacologic treatment.

CHAPTER VIII
SUBSTANCE USE DISORDERS

Items 359-367

Choose the **BEST** response.

359. Each of the following is a valid substance-related diagnosis in DSM-IV **EXCEPT**:

    (A)   substance intoxication
    (B)   substance abuse
    (C)   substance dependence
    (D)   substance-induced organic brain syndrome
    (E)   substance withdrawal

360. Other substance-related DSM-IV diagnoses include

    (A)   substance-induced mood disorder
    (B)   substance-induced sexual dysfunction
    (C)   substance-induced persisting dementia
    (D)   A and C only
    (E)   A, B, and C

361. In general population surveys, what percentage of adults meet criteria for a serious substance-related lifetime diagnosis?

    (A)   4%
    (B)   8%
    (C)   16%
    (D)   25%
    (E)   30%

362. In general population surveys, what percentage of adults meet criteria for a current, serious alcohol-related disorder?

    (A)   2%
    (B)   5%
    (C)   10%
    (D)   18%
    (E)   25%

363. Identify the **TRUE** statement(s) concerning the epidemiology of alcohol-related illness.

    (A)   Men are afflicted up to 4-5 times more than women.
    (B)   Women develop complications more quickly than men.
    (C)   Young adults (age 18-25) have the highest rates of current alcohol-related diagnoses.
    (D)   A and C only
    (E)   A, B, and C

364. Identify the **TRUE** statement(s).

    (A)   Alcohol use contributes to 20 to 50% of all hospital admissions.
    (B)   Alcohol is involved in up to 75% of traffic accidents occurring in the late evening hours.
    (C)   Alcohol is involved in 50% of all homicides and 25% of all suicides.
    (D)   A and C only
    (E)   A, B, and C

365. Choose the appropriate ranking for illicit drugs, from **MOST** to **LEAST** commonly used.

    (A)   marijuana, opioids, prescription drugs, hallucinogens, cocaine
    (B)   prescription drugs, opioids, marijuana, cocaine, hallucinogens
    (C)   marijuana, prescription drugs, cocaine, opioids, hallucinogens
    (D)   cocaine, prescription drugs, marijuana, hallucinogens, opioids
    (E)   prescription drugs, cocaine, marijuana, hallucinogens, opioids

366. People are **MOST** likely to abuse substances that

    (A)   are immediately rewarding to take
    (B)   typically induce tolerance (need for increasing doses to retain their effect)
    (C)   lead to discomfort when withdrawn
    (D)   All of the above
    (E)   None of the above

367. A 35-year-old patient is reluctant to try an antidepressant for fear of becoming a drug addict. The physician should

    (A)   respect her scruples and treat her with psychotherapy alone
    (B)   give her the medication and refer her to a twelve step program
    (C)   reassure her that antidepressants are not drugs of abuse because of oral administration, lack of immediate reward, and lack of tendency to cause tolerance
    (D)   prescribe lower than recommended doses to avoid inducing a "high"
    (E)   explain to the patient she will not become addicted as long as she stops the drug after a few weeks, tapering to avoid withdrawal symptoms

ANSWERS AND TUTORIAL ON ITEMS 359-367

The answers are: **359-D; 360-E; 361-C; 362-B; 363-E; 364-E; 365-C; 366-D; 367-C**. DSM-IV substantially revised the **classification of substance use disorders**. The term substance was chosen to avoid the problems of earlier classifications, for example, the difficulty of distinguishing synthetic ("drugs") and naturally occurring compounds or of basing medical distinctions on differences between legal (nicotine, alcohol, prescribed opioids or amphetamines) and illegal (heroin, marijuana, methamphetamine) chemicals.

The primary substance-related diagnoses in DSM-IV are **substance intoxication**, **withdrawal**, **abuse**, and **dependence**. The particular substance or class of substance (alcohol, amphetamine, cocaine, sedative, inhalant, hallucinogen, PCP like, opioid) is specified if known. The term organic brain syndrome no longer appears. It lacks validity because most major psychiatric syndromes have organic elements, and some brain disorders also have behavioral or psychosocial determinants. Instead, DSM-IV recognizes syndromes in which the effect of a substance on the brain is considered a causal factor by including a substance-related category in the domains of delirium, dementia, mood disorders, anxiety and psychosis. Specifically, DSM-IV provides criteria for **substance-induced psychotic disorder** (with hallucinations or with delusions), **substance-induced mood disorder**, **substance-induced delirium**, **substance-induced anxiety disorder**, **substance-induced persisting dementia**, **substance-induced sexual dysfunction**, **substance-induced sleep disorder**, and **substance-related disorder nos** (not otherwise specified).

Epidemiologically, roughly **16% of people will have a lifetime history of substance abuse or dependence**, with alcohol or alcohol and another substance together accounting for more than two thirds of this number (13%). Simple use is far more common than a use-related diagnosis, at least for legal substances like alcohol. Roughly 85% of people over age 12 admit to some lifetime use of alcohol, 68% to use in the past year and 51% to use in the past month. These figures are higher than, but comparable to, those for cigarettes (73% ever smoked, 32% in the past year and 27% in the past month).

The **rates for use of illicit substances** are: marijuana, 33% ever used, 9.7% current users; cocaine, 11.5% ever used, 0.9% current users; other substances (hallucinogens, inhalants, opioids), ever used 9%, current use <1%. The illicit use of prescribed substances is similar to that of cocaine: 12% ever used; 1.6% current use.

The figures for a **current substance-related diagnosis** are much lower. Roughly 5 to 7% of Americans qualify for an alcohol-related disorder in any given year, with the prevalence rate being 5-6% for men and 1-2% for women. In the case of illicit drugs or a legal drug used improperly, most texts do not differentiate simple use from a use related diagnosis. Any use of an illegal substance is aberrant. Thus, the figures for any use, given above, often appear as prevalence rates for illicit-substance-related diagnoses. Such inflation of prevalence rates masks the fact that some people use illicit substances without developing diagnosable abuse or dependence.

The **epidemiology of alcohol use** shows that men have much higher rates of abuse and dependence than women, although the disease is more variable and rapidly progressive in women. Young adults have higher rates of both alcohol and other substance abuse than either adolescents or older adults.

The staggering **public health consequences of alcohol** and other substance use extend beyond the numbers afflicted with diagnosable substance use disorders. Alcohol use is frequently implicated in cases of spousal and child abuse and incest. It is a contributing cause in all classes of violent death, including car accidents (50-75%), homicide (50%) and suicide (25%). Alcohol is a factor in 20-50% of all hospital admissions. By some measurements, alcohol-related problems are the third leading cause of death in the United States, after cancer and heart disease.

Epidemiologic studies show that alcohol and nicotine, both legal, are by far the most commonly used and abused substances. Marijuana is next, followed by roughly equal use of either prescribed psychoactive drugs or cocaine. The least common drugs of abuse are opioids, inhalants, and hallucinogens.

Drugs can be screened in animals for **abuse potential**. Abusable drugs are rewarding (animals will self-administer them in preference to eating/drinking) and tend to induce both tolerance and withdrawal. The more rapid the onset of the sought for changes, the more likely the drug will be abused. Rapidity of onset is related to the particular drug taken and to the mode of administration. Drugs that are injected or inhaled are especially quick in action. Inhalation, in particular, bypasses first pass metabolism in the liver. Thus, IV use of heroin or snorting of cocaine (especially highly concentrated forms known as crack) quickly leads to abuse.

Conversely, patients may be reassured that most prescribed medications, even psychotropics except benzodiazepines, are not abusable drugs and patients do not become addicted to them. Giving lower doses of antidepressants or prescribing them for a few weeks would be incorrect, since the onset of action is delayed up to three or four weeks and the drugs should be continued for at least four months. (Short courses followed by tapering would be correct for a benzodiazepine). Antidepressants, especially cyclic antidepressants, may precipitate a withdrawal syndrome if stopped abruptly, but this alone does not make them abusable.

Items 368-384

Match the characteristic manifestations of a recent use (intoxication) syndrome in the answers below with the **MOST** appropriate substance in the items. Answers may be used once, more than once, or not at all.

(A)   Euphoria, anxiety, tension, anger or vigilance. Impaired judgement, impaired social or occupational functioning. Two or more of: tachycardia, bradycardia; dilated pupils; elevated or lowered blood pressure; perspiration or chills; nausea/vomiting; agitation/retardation; muscle weakness, respiratory depression, chest pain, cardiac arrhythmia; confusion, seizures, dystonia, coma. May include perceptual disturbances (hallucinations/illusions).

(B)   Belligerence, assaultiveness, impulsiveness, agitation, impaired judgment or functioning. Two or more of: vertical/horizontal nystagmus; numbness, diminished responsiveness to pain; dysarthria; hypertension/tachycardia; hyperacusis; rigidity; seizures or coma. May include hallucinations or illusions.

(C)   Euphoria, followed by apathy/dysphoria; agitation or retardation; impaired judgment or behavior. Pupillary constriction (except in overdose) and one of: drowsiness, slurred speech, impaired attention or memory. May include perceptual disturbances (hallucinations/illusions).

(D)   Euphoria, anxiety, impaired coordination, altered sense of time, impaired judgment, social withdrawal. Two or more of: conjunctival injection, increased appetite, dry mouth, tachycardia. May include perceptual disturbances.

(E)   Inappropriate sexual or aggressive behavior; labile or extreme mood, impaired judgment or functioning. One or more of: slurred speech, incoordination, unsteady gait, nystagmus, impairment of attention or memory, stupor or coma.

(F)   Marked anxiety or depression; ideas of reference; fears of losing one's mind; impaired judgement or functioning and perceptual changes (intensification of perceptions, depersonalization, illusions, hallucinations, synesthesias) and two or more of: pupillary dilatation, tachycardia, sweating, palpitations, blurred vision, tremors, incoordination.

368.   Alcohol

369.   Cocaine

370.   Marijuana (cannabis)

371.   Phencyclidine

372.   Heroin

Select the **BEST** response.

373. All the following have defined intoxication syndromes **EXCEPT**:

   (A)   amphetamines
   (B)   caffeine
   (C)   nicotine
   (D)   cannabis
   (E)   inhalants

374. The psychiatric definition of alcohol intoxication requires

   (A)   a blood alcohol level of 50 mg/dl (.05%)
   (B)   a blood alcohol level of 100 mg/dl (.10%)
   (C)   a blood alcohol level of 250 mg/dl (.25%)
   (D)   only breathalyzer proof of any alcohol use
   (E)   symptoms and behavior

375. The dopaminergic nucleus accumbens is thought to mediate the sensation of reward associated with the use of all the following **EXCEPT**:

   (A)   nicotine
   (B)   cocaine
   (C)   MDMA
   (D)   alcohol
   (E)   opioids

376. Direct suppression of locus ceruleus activity, or indirect suppression via the ventral tegmental area, probably mediates the effects of

   (A)   barbiturates/benzodiazepines
   (B)   alcohol
   (C)   opioids
   (D)   A and C only
   (E)   A, B, and C

377. A 25-year-old man complaining of depression also has nausea, vomiting and diarrhea, dilated pupils, yawning, goose flesh, and insomnia. The substance he recently stopped using is **MOST** likely

(A) alcohol
(B) nicotine
(C) heroin
(D) cocaine
(E) cannabis

378. An 18-year-old woman with depression, exhaustion, vivid dreams, hypersomnia, hyperphagia and sluggishness may be in withdrawal from

(A) cannabis
(B) alcohol
(C) cocaine or amphetamine
(D) opioids
(E) phencyclidine

379. Which drug withdrawal state is **MOST** associated with significant mortality?

(A) alcohol withdrawal delirium (delirium tremens)
(B) amphetamine withdrawal
(C) opioid withdrawal
(D) phencyclidine withdrawal
(E) hallucinogen withdrawal

380. Seizures may occur during

(A) cocaine, phencyclidine or amphetamine intoxication
(B) cannabis intoxication
(C) alcohol or sedative withdrawal
(D) A and C only
(E) A, B, and C

381. Clinically significant withdrawal is **NOT** defined for

(A) hallucinogens
(B) amphetamines
(C) cannabis
(D) A and C only
(E) A, B, and C

382. As defined in DSM-IV, substance **ABUSE** requires maladaptive substance use leading to significant impairment or distress as manifested by

   (A) recurrent use or continued use despite negative consequences (physical hazard, family discord, legal problems, etc.)
   (B) persistent desire for or unsuccessful efforts to cut down this class of substance (craving)
   (C) lifetime history of dependence on this class of substance
   (D) A and C only
   (E) A, B, and C

383. The DSM-IV definition of substance **DEPENDENCE** includes all the following **EXCEPT**:

   (A) tolerance (need for increasing amounts to achieve desired effects)
   (B) withdrawal
   (C) excessive time in drug-seeking activity
   (D) persistent or recurrent use despite physical or psychological complications related to use of this substance
   (E) periods of controlled use, alternating with abstinence or excessive use

384. A 25-year-old civil servant who dropped out of a master's program gives a history of smoking marijuana before and after work and throughout the day most weekends. She stays home to smoke, refusing invitations from friends. She says she can stop anytime she wants to, but, by history, she has stopped only for periods of a few weeks and has always drifted back to her current level of use. She has been told that use of marijuana contributes to her problem with obesity and may have undermined her interest in school. She continues smoking despite professing a desire to lose weight and finish her degree.
   This patient is manifesting

   (A) cannabis intoxication
   (B) cannabis withdrawal
   (C) cannabis abuse
   (D) cannabis dependence
   (E) substance use disorder not otherwise specified

ANSWERS AND TUTORIAL ON ITEMS 368-384

The answers are: **368-E; 369-A; 370-D; 371-B; 372-C; 373-C; 374-E; 375-D; 376-E; 377-C; 378-C; 379-A; 380-D; 381-D; 382-A; 383-E; 384-D. Intoxication** is defined as the characteristic effects of a given substance on physical and psychological functioning. With some drugs, e.g., alcohol, intoxication implies that the person has exceeded a certain threshold or taken an overly large amount of a substance. For others, e.g., hallucinogens, even a minute amount leads to the state described. Psychiatric criteria for intoxication describe symptoms and behavior without regard to measured blood levels or amounts used. The legal definitions of intoxication may require these elements. Thus, a person who becomes excited and violent with a blood alcohol level of 50 mg/dl (a condition once called "pathological intoxication") may be diagnosable as clinically intoxicated but not legally drunk.

The different intoxication syndromes all require significant **maladaptive behavior** or psychological changes that develop during or soon after the use of a substance. Although it causes significant subjective and vegetative changes, nicotine has no defined intoxication syndrome because these changes are not inherently maladaptive. The term intoxication does not capture all the negative consequences of long-term substance use, for example, the carcinogenic or cardiovascular effects of long-term smoking.

Except for a few unique features, e.g. numbness and vertical nystagmus for PCP, reddened eyes and increased appetite for marijuana, and synesthesia for hallucinogens, substances of abuse may have overlapping effects. Clinically, intoxication syndromes are distinguished by the prominence of particular symptoms, unique clustering of symptoms, and associated signs that are not included in the diagnostic criteria. Thus, although perceptual distortions may occur in almost any intoxicated state, if they are the main symptom in someone with marked depersonalization or paranoia but minimal or undetectable changes in heart rate, blood pressure, pupil size and alertness, the most likely substance used is an hallucinogen. Opiates and alcohol both may cause euphoria, incoordination and slurred speech, but can be differentiated by pupillary constriction on the one hand and nystagmus on the other. Associated signs are often extremely helpful but are too variable and unreliable to be part of the definitions. The odor of alcohol or the presence of needle tracks, scars, and abscesses will help the clinician decide if a person is drunk or has been using opiates, even if neither sign is a defining criterion of intoxication.

In Items 368-372, answer F is a description of hallucinogen intoxication. All the others match one of the substances given in the items.

The **overlapping effects** of different substances of abuse, and the tendency of each to lead to compulsive use despite negative consequences, may reflect common mechanisms of brain activity. All stimulants, including nicotine, may enhance the sensation of reward mediated by the dopaminergic nucleus accumbens. Opioids also affect this area. The effects of barbiturates and benzodiazepines, though less clearly worked out, seem to be mediated in part by inhibition of the noradrenergic locus ceruleus. Opioids and possibly alcohol act at the ventral tegmental area, which secondarily suppresses the locus ceruleus. The details of how substances affect receptor function, second messenger systems, and gene expression are still poorly understood.

Many, but not all, substances of abuse produce a **withdrawal state**, with characteristic signs and symptoms. Withdrawal becomes a psychiatric diagnosis when the syndrome produces significant distress or impairment. In general, withdrawal and prolonged abstinence syndromes (defined in DSM-IV as substance-induced mood, anxiety, or sleep disorders) become clinically significant only after prolonged use of a substance. Exceptions do occur; for example, depression and intense craving may occur after only one or two episodes of concentrated cocaine use.

Opioids, sedatives (including alcohol) and stimulants (cocaine, amphetamine) each produce characteristic withdrawal states. **Opioid withdrawal** produces a mixed hypercholinergic and hyperadrenergic picture with dysphoria; nausea, diarrhea and vomiting; piloerection (goose flesh); dilated pupils; lacrimation/rhinorrhea; yawning; fever; muscle aches and insomnia. Brief use of opioids, for example to control postoperative pain, rarely produces significant withdrawal. After prolonged use, by contrast, withdrawal may include persistent dysphoria, insomnia, bradycardia, temperature dysregulation and craving.

Withdrawal from both amphetamines and cocaine produces depression, fatigue, insomnia or hypersomnia with vivid, unpleasant dreams; increased appetite; and agitation or retardation. Most effects are immediate and transient (a few days to a week), though depression, sleep disorder and craving may persist.

Neither stimulant withdrawal nor opioid withdrawal is life-threatening, in the absence of pre-existing, major medical illness. **Alcohol and sedative** (benzodiazepine or barbiturate) **withdrawal**, by contrast, may be fatal, either from recurrent seizures or from cardiovascular collapse after prolonged hyperarousal. In particular, alcohol withdrawal delirium (formerly delirium tremens) has a 5-15% mortality if not treated.

In general **stimulant intoxication** resembles sedative withdrawal. Either may cause extreme hyperarousal, including seizures. Stimulant intoxication only partially reverses sedative intoxication, despite the opposing effects of the two classes of drugs. A person who tries to reverse the effective of alcohol or benzodiazepines with caffeine, amphetamines, or cocaine will still be dangerously drunk and incapacitated, even if subjectively more alert.

Clinically significant withdrawal is not a necessary element of substance abuse or dependence. Cannabis, hallucinogens, and inhalants do not produce recognizable withdrawal syndromes (except possibly desire for continued use or craving).

Intoxication and withdrawal both relate to the immediate effects of substance use or cessation of use. Longer-term patterns of substance use are classified as either abuse or dependence. Abuse requires only one manifestation of impairment or distress, specifically failure to fulfill major role obligations; recurrent substance use that is physically hazardous (driving while intoxicated); recurrent substance-related legal problems, or continued use despite persistent or recurrent problems caused by the substance. Patients who abuse drugs may lack the desire to cut down, but in theory, they are able to so. Those who are substance-dependent, by contrast, try and repeatedly fail to reduce or stop using. By current definition, substance abuse cannot be diagnosed if the person has ever met criteria for dependence on the same class of substance.

Dependence, the more severe substance-related diagnosis, implies three of 7 criteria: tolerance (need for increasing amounts or decreased effect of the same amount); withdrawal; recurrent unintentional overuse; inability to cut down or control use; inordinate time given to obtaining, using, or recovering from use of a substance (drug-seeking behavior); reduction in important work, social or recreational activities; and continued use despite persistent or recurrent problems related to the substance.

Although physiological tolerance and withdrawal are often a feature of substance dependence, they are not essential--a cannabis abuser who spends a large percentage of his or her time intoxicated, uses more than intended on numerous occasions, can't voluntarily stop using, and has dropped out of school would be diagnosable as cannabis-dependent. In general, however, drugs with the greatest likelihood of inducing tolerance and withdrawal (stimulants, sedatives/alcohol, and opiates) are most likely to induce dependence. Once a person has met criteria for dependence, if he or she begins to use the same substance, the diagnosis would be relapse rather than abuse of that substance.

Items 385-390

Choose the **BEST** response.

385.   Sixty-five percent of women and seventy six percent of men with alcohol abuse or dependence have an additional psychiatric diagnosis. The **MOST** common comorbid diagnosis in patients with alcohol-related problems is

    (A)   major depressive disorder
    (B)   social phobia
    (C)   abuse of another substance
    (D)   antisocial personality disorder
    (E)   dysthymic disorder

386.   The suicide rate in patients with alcohol-related disorders is

    (A)   2%
    (B)   8%
    (C)   10%
    (D)   15%
    (E)   the same as the rate in the general population

387.   All of the following are components of the CAGE screening test for alcohol abuse **EXCEPT**:

    (A)   need for an eye-opener
    (B)   guilt over alcohol use
    (C)   felt need to cut down on drinking
    (D)   angry outbursts related to drinking
    (E)   feeling annoyed by others' criticism of drinking

388. Physical findings in alcoholics may include

    (A)   spider angiomata of the face, enlarged or shrunken liver, peripheral neuropathy, cerebellar dysfunction
    (B)   macrocytic or microcytic anemia
    (C)   elevated γ-glutamyl transpeptidase (GTT)
    (D)   A and C only
    (E)   A, B, and C

389. Type I alcoholism differs from Type II in

    (A)   typical age of onset (adult vs. childhood or adolescence)
    (B)   personality traits (guilt, worry, introversion vs. impulsivity, distractibility, restlessness)
    (C)   lack of prominent family history, better response to treatment
    (D)   All of the above
    (E)   None of the above

390. The ratio of Type I to Type II alcoholism is

    (A)   1:1
    (B)   1:2
    (C)   2:1
    (D)   3:1
    (E)   3:2

ANSWERS AND TUTORIAL ON ITEMS 385-390

The answers are: **385-C; 386-D; 387-D; 388-E; 389-D; 390-D**. More is known about **alcohol use disorders** and their treatment than about other substances of abuse. Alcohol-related diagnoses occur in isolation only 25-35% of the time. The most common comorbid diagnosis is abuse of or dependence on another substance. Depression, dysthymia and anxiety disorders, especially social phobia, may precede the onset of alcohol use, suggesting that a desire for self-medication incites use in some people. Antisocial personality occurs in a high percentage (35-60%) of those who use illicit substances and to a lesser degree in alcoholics, especially Type II alcoholics (see below). This association reflects both the effect of substances on the brain systems that mediate social behavior and the ineffectiveness of legal proscription against drugs of abuse on those with premorbid antisocial traits.

    Although not the most common comorbid diagnosis in those who abuse alcohol or other substances, **depression**, which occurs in about 30% of opioid users and 40% of alcoholics at some point in their lives, is of great clinical significance because of the associated risk of suicide. Chronic alcohol abusers have a 15% suicide rate which is roughly 20 times that of the general population.

The four item **CAGE test** is a highly sensitive, quick screen for alcohol abuse in men. The acronym reminds the interviewer to ask if the person has ever 1. Felt the need to **C**ut down on drinking? 2. Felt **A**nnoyed by criticisms of drinking? 3. Felt **G**uilty about drinking? 4. Taken a morning **E**ye-opener? A single positive response suggests possible alcohol abuse and should lead to careful follow-up questions about the effects of drinking on the person's interpersonal relationships and general functioning.

Patients with **alcohol dependence** may have a variety of objective findings. These include signs of liver disease (angiomata, palmar erythema, fatty enlargement of the liver or shrinkage from cirrhosis, abnormal liver function tests); macrocytic anemia and signs of peripheral neuropathy from folate deficiency; microcytic anemia from chronic occult GI bleeding; and cardiomyopathy. GTT is a sensitive marker of alcohol abuse, though relatively nonspecific. The combination of elevated GTT with elevated MCV (macrocytosis) correctly identifies up to 90% of alcohol-dependent patients.

Those who misuse alcohol may be subclassified as **Type I** or **Type II** alcoholics. Type I, which accounts for 75% of all alcoholic patients, is defined by adult onset; introverted, dependent personality features; equal prevalence in males and females; relatively little family history and better response to treatment. Type II, which accounts for only 25% of patients, corresponds more to the stereotype of an alcoholic. Males predominate; most have a strongly positive family history. Type II alcoholics typically begin drinking in adolescence or even childhood. These patients are impulsive, distractible, restless and relatively refractory to treatment.

Items 391-395

A 40-year-old, married man is brought to the emergency room following a car accident. His blood alcohol level is 250 mg/dl and his urine toxicology screen reveals recent use of cocaine. His wife reports that he drinks daily, beginning when he wakes up, and uses cocaine in binges on the weekends. He has shown this pattern of substance use on a continuous basis for the past four years. He requires hospital admission for injuries suffered in the accident.

391.   The initial hospital treatment should include

(A)   administration of thiamine in his IV fluid
(B)   treatment of cocaine withdrawal with sustained release methylphenidate
(C)   treatment of alcohol withdrawal with careful hydration and a tapering schedule of benzodiazepines
(D)   A and C only
(E)   A, B, and C

392. Once the patient has been detoxified, treatment should include

    (A)   assessment of his level of understanding of his substance-related problem
    (B)   referral to professional psychoeducational groups, plus self-help
    (C)   meetings with him and his wife together, to enlist her in supporting his sobriety
    (D)   A and C only
    (E)   A, B, and C

393. Once detoxified, the patient shows signs of depression, with dysphoria, fatigue, hopelessness, insomnia, poor concentration, and passive suicidal ideation without intent. Initiation of antidepressant treatment should

    (A)   occur immediately
    (B)   be deferred for one week, until cocaine withdrawal is complete
    (C)   be deferred for four weeks, to see if symptoms remit with abstinence from alcohol
    (D)   be deferred six months, until patient is firmly invested in self-help
    (E)   not occur, as the patient is likely to abuse the drugs prescribed

394. Which of the following would indicate the need for inpatient admission for substance abuse

    (A)   repeated failure to detoxify as an outpatient
    (B)   a comorbid major psychiatric diagnosis such as psychosis or depression with suicidal ideation
    (C)   a comorbid medical condition that might make withdrawal dangerous to the patient
    (D)   All of the above
    (E)   None of the above

395. After six months of sobriety, alcohol-dependent patients

    (A)   return to controlled social drinking in 10% of cases
    (B)   return to controlled social drinking in up to 30% of cases
    (C)   return to controlled social drinking only if maintained on naltrexone
    (D)   return to controlled social drinking only if maintained on disulfiram
    (E)   almost always relapse if they try to return to controlled social drinking under any conditions

ANSWERS AND TUTORIAL ON ITEMS 391-395

The answers are: **391-D; 392-E; 393-C; 394-D; 395-E.** In the hospital, this patient will withdraw from both alcohol and cocaine. Only the **alcohol withdrawal** is medically serious. The patient is at risk for developing acute encephalopathy if given glucose without thiamine. In addition, he needs to be given fluids and a benzodiazepine to prevent alcohol withdrawal delirium (or seizures). Alternate agents such as carbamazepine or α- or β-blockers are used in detoxification protocols in some settings, but the current recommended method is to place the person on a tapering schedule of a cross-tolerant sedative. Benzodiazepines have replaced barbiturates, chloral hydrate, and paraldehyde for this purpose.

Efforts to treat this man for substance abuse will not succeed if he does not recognize that he is ill. Initially, the physician needs to determine whether or not he admits to the problem. After a serious event like a car accident, people who have been "in denial" may become willing to accept their diagnosis. If not, being able to confront a patient with medical evidence of substance abuse may help. Patients then need to learn about the many different presentations of substance misuse, the social and medical consequences of continued use, and various forms of treatment. Psychoeducational groups can provide much of this information and be a bridge to consistent participation in self-help. When a family member is available, involving that person in treatment is essential. Family members need to learn to recognize and change ways they may protect the patient from the consequences of substance abuse ("enabling"), so that the person will be more motivated to remain abstinent. The family members of substance abusers also need to be evaluated for psychiatric problems. Depression and substance abuse are commonly found in people close to the abusing patient. Such problems can cause a partner to subvert a patient's recovery if both are not treated concurrently.

Withdrawal from cocaine mimics major depression, but would typically improve within a week of cessation of use. Long-term alcohol users may also exhibit symptoms of depression in the early phases of sobriety. It takes about a month for the immediate physical effects of drinking to subside. When to prescribe an antidepressant is a matter of clinical judgment, but it is reasonable to initiate treatment if symptoms persist after a month of no drug use. Adequate treatment for depression will likely enhance the patient's motivation to participate in self-help and maintain sobriety. Patients almost never abuse antidepressants, which can therefore be given safely to abstinent substance abusers.

When possible, **substance detoxification** should occur on an outpatient basis. Patients who are detoxified in a setting where the environmental cues associated with use are absent may relapse quickly when released. Intensive outpatient treatment during the withdrawal/detoxification phase helps people substitute treatment resources (clinic staff or self-help) for substance use while in their natural environment. Inpatient detoxification is still indicated for patients with complicating medical illness, repeated failure to detoxify as outpatients, or a serious comorbid psychiatric diagnosis, especially if the patient is at risk for suicide.

Returned to **controlled social use** of a substance is almost never possible for substance-dependent persons. Naltrexone, which may reduce the extent and severity of relapses in alcoholics who drink in a binge fashion, does not permit a return to controlled drinking.

Disulfiram, which causes symptoms of toxicity when a person drinks alcohol, is incompatible with drinking at any level. Sustained, complete abstinence is the goal of all treatment for all substance-dependent persons.

Items 396 and 397

A 60-year-old woman comes to the physician's office complaining of unsteadiness and a burning sensation in her feet. She reports that she is under a lot of stress, because her husband is threatening divorce. On closer questioning, she admits the issue is that he thinks she drinks too much. Her neurological examination reveals apparent loss of position and vibratory sense in stocking distribution in both lower extremities with intact reflexes, muscle strength, cerebellar functions and cranial nerves. On mental status examination she seems mildly anxious, and some of her answers are rambling. She is oriented to place, year and day of the week but not date. She claims she can't do serial subtractions because she is not good in math. She remembers two of three objects at five minutes, can recall 5 digits forward and 3 in reverse. She then refuses the rest of the mental status examination.

396. The **MOST** likely diagnosis is

   (A)   conversion disorder
   (B)   dementia secondary to alcohol-induced hypocalcemia
   (C)   alcohol-induced anxiety disorder
   (D)   folate deficiency

397. Immediately available laboratory screening will show

   (A)   normal CBC, elevated sedimentation rate
   (B)   Hgb 10.3 gm/100 ml (nl=12-16 gm/100 ml); HCT 32% (nl 37-47%); MCV 79 fL (nl=82-92); MCHC 30% (nl=32-36%) (microcytic anemia)
   (C)   Hgb 10.3 gm/ml (nl=12-16 gm/ml); HCT 34% (nl=37-47%); MCV 101 fL (nl=82-92); MCHC=33% (nl=32-36%) (macrocytic anemia)
   (D) Na^+ 139 mEq/L (nl 135-145) K^+ 3.4 mEq/l (nl=3.5-5.5) Cl^- 99 mEq/l (nl=98-106); HCO_3^- 18 mEq/l (nl=26-28); Anion gap=25 (Nl <15)

ANSWERS AND TUTORIAL ON ITEMS 396 AND 397

The answers are: **396-D; 397-C**. Various clinically significant nutritional deficiencies and metabolic imbalances occur in **alcoholics**, affecting many parts of the nervous system and producing different mental status changes. Deficiencies of folate and vitamin B_{12}, which may co-occur, can cause **macrocytic anemia, peripheral neuropathy**, delirium or dementia. This patient has the classic loss of position and vibratory sense seen in peripheral neuropathy, macrocytic anemia, and subtle mental status changes characteristic of early dementia.

The patient's normal reflexes are evidence against the deficiency of Ca^{2+} or Mg^{2+} which can occur in alcoholics and lead to delirium, psychosis, hyperreflexia, tetany, seizures, and death. Although this patient does not have symptoms consistent with ketoacidosis, it would be important to screen for this by measuring electrolytes, since alcoholics can develop ketoacidosis from alcohol, malnutrition, or from diabetes mellitus secondary to destruction of the pancreas.

Symptoms are often difficult to detect in intoxicated patients, and uncooperative behavior, even when the patient is sober, often leads medical professionals to perform cursory or inadequate medical evaluation. Physicians are quick to apply pejorative psychiatric labels to alcoholic patients. While stocking and glove anesthesia or paresthesia are sometimes symptoms of hyperventilation or conversion disorder, burning sensations and a stocking distribution of the loss of position and vibratory sense are typical of peripheral neuropathy. Alcoholics suffer neuropathy both from alcohol itself and from associated vitamin deficiencies. Detection and differentiation of various alcohol-related neurological dysfunctions is crucial, since many have specific remedies. Left untreated, vitamin deficiency, electrolyte abnormalities, ketoacidosis or diabetes mellitus can lead to permanent, incapacitating neurological damage, even death.

CHAPTER IX
ANXIETY, SOMATOFORM, DISSOCIATIVE, EATING, AND PERSONALITY DISORDERS

Items 398-404

Match the specific disorder in the answers below with the **BEST** descriptive phrase concerning that disorder in the items. Answers may be used once, more than once, or not at all.

- (A) Somatization disorder
- (B) Panic disorder with agoraphobia
- (C) Generalized anxiety disorder
- (D) Somatoform disorder
- (E) Posttraumatic stress disorder
- (F) Social phobia
- (G) Brief psychotic disorder
- (H) Borderline personality disorder
- (I) Panic disorder without agoraphobia
- (J) Acute stress disorder

398. Intense anxiety stimulated by perceived abandonment or mistreatment by important people.

399. Fears of dying, going crazy or losing control, associated with signs of autonomic arousal, and avoidance of situations from which escape might be difficult or help unavailable during an episode.

400. Uncontrollable, excessive worry about a variety of events or activities, occurring more days than not for at least six months. Associated symptoms of muscle tension, sleep disturbance, and decreased concentration.

401. Three months of intrusive recollections following an experience of intense fear and horror in the face of threatened or actual severe injury or death. Avoidance of stimuli that bring the event to mind, emotional detachment, sleep disorder, poor concentration, and exaggerated startle response.

402. Many physical complaints, including pain, sexual dysfunction, gastrointestinal distress, and inexplicable neurological symptoms.

403. History of sexual or physical abuse in childhood. Difficulty with dysphoria, anxiety, and anger. Self-mutilation to relieve painful numbness and emptiness.

404. Intense anxiety or panic in situations associated with fears of being humiliated or embarrassed. Predisposing condition for alcohol abuse.

ANSWERS AND TUTORIAL ON ITEMS 398-404

The answers are: **398-H; 399-B; 400-C; 401-E; 402-A; 403-H; 404-F.** DSM-IV assigns separate categories to anxiety disorders, personality disorders, somatoform disorders, and dissociative disorders. It is important to recognize that **anxiety as a symptom** appears in many psychiatric disorders in and outside of these categories. Thus, anxiety may figure prominently in somatization disorder; all forms of psychotic disorder including brief psychotic disorder and schizophrenia; major depressions; avoidant, dependent, and borderline personality disorders; and stimulant intoxication or sedative withdrawal, among other common psychiatric problems.

All clinically significant forms of anxiety involve a mental state of **dread or fear** and somatic manifestations (e.g., palpitations, churning stomach, diarrhea, urge to urinate, restlessness, sleep problems, and muscle tension). In the anxiety disorders, these symptoms, by definition, lead to significant functional impairment.

Differentiating among the **anxiety disorders** requires classification of the patient's most prominent anxiety as persistent, as in generalized anxiety disorder, or brief and intense, as in panic disorder, social phobia, and simple phobia. Sometimes distinguishing different patterns of anxiety is impossible. Bouts of acute, severe symptoms can occur superimposed on the persistent, diffuse symptoms of generalized anxiety disorder. Between acute episodes, patients with mainly brief anxiety states may have persistent fear of their symptoms (anticipatory anxiety). Recognizing which aspect of the anxiety is most prominent and disabling requires clinical experience. If several different patterns of anxiety co-exist, two or more anxiety disorders may be diagnosed concurrently. Indeed, among the anxiety disorders, comorbidity is common.

The characteristic themes or **triggers** of patients' anxiety also help distinguish one anxiety disorder from another. In **generalized anxiety**, patients have fears concerning many aspects of their personal security, typically, money, health, the welfare of family members, and so on. In **panic disorder**, patients fear the experience of panic itself. Those who also avoid situations that they believe might trigger a panic attack, or where it would be dangerous or embarrassing to have a panic attack, are classified as having panic disorder with **agoraphobia**.

Patients with **social phobia** fear humiliation, scrutiny or rejection in interactions with others, sometimes only strangers, sometimes only in possible intimate relationships. These patients avoid the social situations they fear, for example, by limiting the kind of work they will do or by being unable to form close attachments. Many will use alcohol to make threatening situations bearable. This pattern can progress to the development of frank alcohol abuse or dependence. The early identification and treatment of social phobia is an extremely important task, as it may prevent later alcohol-related problems.

Traumatic events, by definition, are events which evoke intense fear and horror in situations where the person feels helpless and endangered. People respond to such events in many ways. Those who use dissociation, a trance-like state that separates the events from the associated painful emotions, are most at risk to develop **acute stress disorder**. This disorder, by definition, subsides within a month. A mixed pattern of anxiety and dissociative symptoms that persist longer would be classified as **posttraumatic stress disorder** (PTSD). The cardinal feature of PTSD is intrusive reliving of the trauma in forced recollection, nightmares, or flashbacks. Intrusive symptoms typically erupt through a state of numbness, loss of interest, feelings of inability to relate normally to others, and a changed view of the future. The chief precipitant to anxiety in PTSD, then, is the welling up of unpleasant emotions related to a past traumatic event. Patients with PTSD also have symptoms of chronic hyperarousal, including sleep disruptions, irritability, low threshold for startle, hypervigilance, physical reactivity to reminders, and diminished concentration.

People with **borderline personality disorder** typically have problems soothing themselves and maintaining a consistent sense of their own identity either when alone or when involved in close relationships. Thus, the main precipitant to their often severe anxiety is disruption in relationships that sustain their shaky equilibrium. Even minor separations, for example, can precipitate severe reactions. Classical psychoanalytic understanding of borderline personality "explains" this anxiety by analogizing it to the anxiety experienced by a two- or three-year-old child negotiating the stage of separation/individuation. This theory postulates that parental failure to encourage and support separation/individuation impairs the patient's sense of self and ability to regulate anxiety. More recent research suggests that borderline personality results from much more severe failures of parenting. Thus, 60-80% of patients with borderline personality disorder report experiencing abuse, especially sexual abuse, during childhood. Having been overstimulated or constantly vigilant in childhood, borderline patients develop high anxiety but cannot learn from trusted adults how to sooth and contain their feelings. Moreover, many preborderline children were abused at the stage when they were dependent on adults for basic survival. The threat of separation thus triggers not anxiety, but panic.

In addition to anxiety, borderline patients have symptoms similar to the numbing seen in those with PTSD, including painful feelings of emptiness. Cutting, burning and other forms of self-mutilation, as well as suicidal gestures and attempts, are a cardinal feature of this disorder and are often explained by the patient as the only available means of coping with anxiety and emptiness.

Somatization disorder, though classified under **somatoform disorders**, overlaps with the anxiety disorders. In both, patients typically seek medical attention for cryptic physical symptoms. The symptoms of anxiety disorders are usually readily explainable as manifestations of autonomic arousal. Most anxious patients will, if asked, also be able to describe their fearful mental state. In somatization disorder, the symptoms are more varied and more difficult to explain. By definition, the patient complains of problems in at least four different organ systems--usually gastrointestinal, neurologic, urogenital, and cardiorespiratory. No clear physical basis for the complaints can be found. Often people with this disorder deny anxiety or psychic distress except for distress about their physical condition. The cause of somatization disorder is unknown. The disorder, which is most common in women, aggregates in families where there appears to be genetic risk for antisocial personality disorder in men.

Items 405-414

Match the drugs used to treat certain disorders or symptom patterns in the items with the drugs that are **MOST** appropriately used to treat these disorders in the answers below. Answers may be used once, more than once, or not at all.

      (A)   Thioridazine, alprazolam, propranolol
      (B)   Serotonin-specific reuptake inhibitors (SSRIs), monoamine oxidase inhibitors (MAOIs), desipramine, alprazolam/clonazepam
      (C)   SSRIs, clomipramine
      (D)   Alprazolam buspirone, propranolol
      (E)   Buspirone, benzodiazepines, imipramine
      (F)   Clomipramine, thioridazine, propranolol
      (G)   Propranolol, atenolol

405.   Panic attacks

406.   Generalized anxiety

407.   Performance anxiety

408.   Obsessive-compulsive disorder

Choose the **BEST** response.

409.   Pharmacotherapy alone is insufficient treatment for anxiety because

      (A)   Available drugs lack efficacy.
      (B)   Drugs have little effect on avoidance behaviors.
      (C)   Available drugs have unacceptably high levels of toxicity, including lethality in overdose.
      (D)   A and C only
      (E)   A, B, and C

410. The percentage of the general population that uses benzodiazepines annually (other than as sleeping pills) is

(A)   3%
(B)   11%
(C)   20%
(D)   35%

411. Phenothiazines, thiothixenes, and butyrophenones are **POOR** choices for the treatment of primary anxiety disorders because

(A)   They lack antianxiety effects.
(B)   They have long-term toxicities not associated with other available drugs.
(C)   They are unacceptably dangerous in overdoses, which are a particular risk for anxious patients who are also depressed.
(D)   A and C only
(E)   A, B, and C

412. In the treatment of anxiety, all the following have a delayed onset of action and, indeed, may increase anxiety initially **EXCEPT**:

(A)   fluoxetine
(B)   phenelzine
(C)   desipramine
(D)   lorazepam
(E)   sertraline

413. The likelihood that a person will abuse a benzodiazepine given for anxiety

(A)   is mainly a factor of the half-life of the drug
(B)   is highest in older patients
(C)   is low except in alcoholics, recovered alcoholics, and first degree relatives of alcoholics
(D)   A and C only
(E)   A, B, and C

414. Although it is a modified cyclic antidepressant, clomipramine is generally **NOT** given for conditions other than obsessive-compulsive disorder because

(A)   Its anticholinergic side-effects are severe and unacceptable to most patients.
(B)   It lacks efficacy in other conditions.
(C)   It also has extrapyramidal side-effects.
(D)   A and C only
(E)   A, B, and C

ANSWERS AND TUTORIAL ON ITEMS 405-414

The answers are: **405-B; 406-E; 407-G; 408-C; 409-B; 410-B; 411-B; 412-D; 413-C; 414-A**. When side-effects and therapeutic effects are balanced against each other, the best tolerated anxiolytic antidepressants appear to be the **MAOIs** and the **SSRIs**, especially for acute, intense anxiety, as seen in panic, social phobia, and posttraumatic stress disorder. Systematic research has shown that the MAOIs and imipramine/desipramine are effective against various forms of anxiety, including panic. Increasing evidence also supports the broad anxiolytic properties of the SSRIs. Because these antidepressants also induce anxiety and all require three to four weeks to bring about a therapeutic response (**response latency**), patients may not tolerate them, especially if used alone. The benzodiazepine receptor agonists alprazolam, clonazepam, and lorazepam are all effective against panic and have an immediate onset of action. Physicians initially often prescribe combinations of antidepressants and benzodiazepines and then wean the patient from the latter after a few weeks so as to minimize the potential for dependence and abuse.

The treatment of anxiety disorders usually requires a combination of specialized psychotherapy and psychotropic drugs. Drug therapy has improved markedly in recent decades, and effective drugs with limited side-effects, minimal toxicity, and safety in overdose are currently available. While drug treatment often brings substantial symptomatic relief, however, drugs alone may not reverse the patient's functional disability, which usually involves avoidance of anxiety-producing situations.

The availability of a wide variety of drugs to relieve anxiety is of great benefit to patients as shown by the statistic that 11% of the general population annually uses a benzodiazepine for purposes other than as a hypnotic.

Thioridazine, like all antipsychotic drugs (i.e., phenothiazines/butyrophenones--dopamine receptor antagonists) has marked anxiolytic properties, especially for the intense anxiety seen in the prodromal and active phases of psychosis. Most antipsychotic drugs are safe in overdose. However, all dopamine receptor antagonists produce significant extrapyramidal or anticholinergic side-effects. All except clozapine and related atypical agents pose the long-term risk of tardive dyskinesia, an irreversible and disfiguring neurologic condition. The availability of effective, safer alternatives makes the dopamine receptor antagonists unacceptable for anxiety except anxiety related to psychosis.

All classes of antidepressants (SSRIs, MAOIs, cyclic antidepressants, trazodone, nefazodone, and venlafaxine) relieve anxiety in depressed patients. SSRIs, cyclic antidepressants, and MAOIs also may be used in patients who are anxious but not depressed. Paradoxically, the antidepressants most commonly given to relieve anxiety (fluoxetine, sertraline, phenelzine, desipramine) can also stimulate it. Treatment-related increases in anxiety tend to occur early when synaptic levels of neurotransmitters rise before compensatory changes occur in receptor sensitivities.

Except in alcoholics, sedative abusers, and people with first degree relatives who are alcoholics, the likelihood of **benzodiazepine dependence** or abuse is generally low if the drugs are prescribed for less than four months in a row.

β-adrenergic receptor blockers (propranolol/atenolol and related drugs) may relieve some of the peripheral manifestations of a panic attack but do not affect the core experience of terror. Thus, β-blockers are generally not useful in panic disorder.

While ineffective in the treatment of panic, **buspirone**, which is active at 5-HT_{1A}, 5-HT_2 and D_2 receptors, is useful in the treatment of generalized anxiety. It lacks the dependence/abuse problems of the benzodiazepine receptor agonists, partly because, like the antidepressants, it produces relief over a period of 3 to 6 weeks, but not immediately. Benzodiazepine receptor agonists also may relieve generalized anxiety symptoms. Since generalized anxiety disorder, by current definition, lasts at least six months, the likelihood that patients will become dependent because of persistent use is substantial. Nevertheless, maintenance on a benzodiazepine may be preferable to persistent, disabling generalized anxiety. When generalized anxiety exists in the context of a major depression, it tends to respond to antidepressant treatment. Thus, all three types of drugs are of use in the treatment of this symptom pattern.

Performance anxiety (stage fright or social phobia in performance situations) is the only type of anxiety that reliably responds to β-adrenergic receptor blockers alone. These drugs lack the potential for dependence, tolerance or abuse. In the low doses (20-80 mg) required for relief of performance anxiety, they also produce minimal side-effects. Why performance anxiety responds so well to these drugs while other anxiety does not is a mystery.

SSRIs and **clomipramine** in high doses are the preferred treatment for **obsessive-compulsive symptoms**. Other antianxiety and antidepressant drugs are much less effective for this problem. While it is an effective antidepressant, clomipramine has a very unfavorable anticholinergic/antihistaminic side-effect profile. For this reason, it is used only for obsessive-compulsive disorder. It is becoming the second choice drug, even for this condition, because the SSRIs are so much better tolerated (though not quite as effective).

Items 415-417

A 27-year-old female graduate student seeks treatment at the university health service for dizziness, palpitations, and pressure in her chest. During these spells, which last for five to ten minutes at a time, she fears she will faint or even die. She takes a circuitous route to school to avoid crossing large streets, where previous episodes have occurred, because she fears being run over if she faints. She avoids classes where she might be called upon to speak. She finds that staying up late to finish papers makes attacks more frequent, and she is having trouble completing assignments. She once took her pulse during an episode and reports it was 100 bpm.

415. The **MOST** likely diagnosis is

 (A)   somatization disorder
 (B)   panic disorder with agoraphobia
 (C)   paroxysmal atrial tachycardia
 (D)   hypoglycemia
 (E)   specific phobia

416. After a normal physical examination, further medical evaluation of her symptoms

    (A)   is unwarranted
    (B)   should include a glucose tolerance test
    (C)   should include CBC, serum electrolytes, fasting glucose, thyroid function tests, and urine toxicology
    (D)   should include Holter monitor and an echocardiogram for mitral valve prolapse
    (E)   should include TRH stimulation test and dexamethasone-suppression test

417. Treatment may involve all the following **EXCEPT**:

    (A)   psychoeducation
    (B)   cognitive exercises to change her catastrophic appraisal of her symptoms
    (C)   encouragement to expose herself to the situations she is avoiding
    (D)   buspirone/propranolol
    (E)   SSRI, alprazolam

ANSWERS AND TUTORIAL ON ITEMS 415-417

The answers are: **415-B; 416-C; 417-D**. The patient displays all the elements of **panic disorder**. She describes intense but brief anxiety episodes with both bodily symptoms and exaggerated beliefs about the dangers of an attack. In addition, one can infer that she experiences fear of the attacks (anticipatory anxiety). She avoids situations that might be embarrassing in the face of panic, from which escape might be difficult, or help unavailable (agoraphobia).

Although patients with panic disorder and patients with **somatization disorder** are both concerned about physical symptoms, by definition, somatization disorder includes symptoms in four different clusters: pain, gastrointestinal dysfunction, sexual dysfunction, and pseudoneurological dysfunction. The occasional confusion between the two diagnoses may reflect the fact that both panic disorder and somatization disorder show a female predominance (2 or 3:1 for panic disorder; 5:1 for somatization disorder) and tend to present in young adulthood. Panic disorder is more common than somatization disorder (1.5 to 3 percent in the general population, rather than 0.5 percent).

Paroxysmal atrial tachycardia (PAT) is not necessarily accompanied by intense subjective anxiety. It requires the characteristic doubling of the pulse rate and EKG evidence for diagnosis. Hypoglycemia rarely induces severe panic or anticipatory anxiety, except in the case of an insulin reaction. Patients are generally sweaty and hungry during an episode.

Specific phobias, by definition, involve reactions to discreet cues or situations, typically animals, aspects of the natural environment, blood/injection/injury, planes, elevators or enclosed places. The phobic stimulus may trigger a panic attack and avoidance, but only of the specific feared situation.

The **medical evaluation** of a person with **panic disorder** is influenced by the person's age and general health. Simple screening for physical factors that may present with symptoms of noradrenergic effects (arousal) generally focuses on conditions that have a significant likelihood of appearing in young people, especially young women. These factors include anemia, hyperthyroidism, and substance abuse (either stimulant use or alcohol/sedative withdrawal). These conditions are diagnosed by history, physical examination, bloodwork, and urine toxicology. Electrolyte deficiencies, especially hypocalcemia, may also produce anxiety.

More extensive work-ups are indicated only if the patient has an unusual symptom or finding or does not respond to treatment. For example, if a click murmur is found, more extensive work-up for mitral valve prolapse, with echocardiogram and EKG, may be indicated. However, such studies are not routine. Indeed, the association between panic disorder and mitral valve prolapse may be not causal but coincidental, related to the tendency of both conditions to present in young women. In the absence of insulin use, hypoglycemia, even if present, is also often merely an incidental finding--that is, patients may show low glucose levels when they are not experiencing panic and may have normal glucose levels during a panic attack. Thus, a glucose tolerance test is not used in screening. The TRH stimulation test and dexamethasone-suppression tests are of research interest in the evaluation of depression, especially with melancholic features, but are not relevant in panic disorder.

The prevailing **psychotherapeutic approach** to panic disorder with agoraphobia is cognitive behavioral therapy. Its core elements are psychoeducation, relaxation, changes in cognitive appraisal of the anxiety and the situations that provoke it, and gradual exposure to feared situations. Psychoeducation involves teaching people that anxiety, even panic, is an intrinsic physiological mechanism designed to protect the person in dangerous situations (the "fight or flight response") and not, in itself, dangerous. Relaxation exercises teach patients that they have the power to bring on a sense of relaxation, just as they have the power to bring on panic. Patients are encouraged to use relaxation and controlled breathing techniques as they expose themselves to the situations they fear. After prolonged exposure, with or without experiencing the anxiety, future vulnerability to panic in the same situation diminishes markedly. Changes in cognition--relinquishing the belief that panic symptoms are dangerous or will result in loss of control--follow from educational sessions, from specific techniques that challenge catastrophic beliefs, and from successful exposure. Alprazolam and SSRIs, but not buspirone or propranolol, are also common elements of the treatment of panic disorder.

Items 418-425

Choose the **BEST** response.

418. Somatization, a term connoting complaints of bodily illness in place of psychological distress

    (A)   Is often motivated by conscious or unconscious desire for the privileges of the sick role.
    (B)   Is often learned in childhood environments where other means of coping with psychological distress are unavailable.
    (C)   Occurs in families where illness is rewarded with unusual degrees of nurturance and care or other family members somaticize or are chronically ill.
    (D)   A and C only
    (E)   A, B, and C

419. Other factors encouraging somatization include all of the following **EXCEPT**:

    (A)   Cultural norms that accept physical but not psychological grounds for illness or disability.
    (B)   Insufficient ability to express emotion in language, due to immature or deficient language skills.
    (C)   Societies that discriminate against mental illnesses, psychological or behavioral problems in allowing for social benefits (insurance, pensions, etc.).
    (D)   Oversupply of specialized, technological medical resources.
    (E)   Personal experience of severe trauma, especially when emotions related to the trauma are difficult to remember or express in words.

420. Somatization as a coping mechanism is a **PROMINENT** feature of

    (A)   conversion disorder
    (B)   histrionic personality disorder
    (C)   pain disorder
    (D)   A and C only
    (E)   A, B, and C

421. Somatization disorder

    (A)   Requires one or more each of pain, gastrointestinal symptoms, sexual symptoms, and pseudoneurological symptoms not readily explained by a medical condition.

    (B)   Can begin at any time in life, usually following a major life event or traumatic experience.

    (C)   Cannot be diagnosed with sufficient reliability to be studied epidemiologically.

    (D)   A and C only

    (E)   A, B, and C.

422. Patients who display symptoms that suggest a medical or neurological illness but have no physiological basis for their problems may be suffering from

    (A)   conversion disorder

    (B)   pain disorder

    (C)   malingering

    (D)   A and C only

    (E)   A, B, and C

423. If the symptom(s) are of discreet onset, are not intentionally produced and appear to be associated with some psychological factor, either a significant stressor or some irresolvable conflict, the **MOST** likely diagnosis is

    (A)   conversion disorder

    (B)   factitious disorder

    (C)   malingering

    (D)   Munchausen's syndrome

    (E)   body dysmorphic disorder

424. In the absence of another major psychiatric syndrome, excessive concern about having serious medical illness that cannot be relieved by appropriate medical reassurance is called

    (A)   malingering

    (B)   hypochondriasis

    (C)   somatic obsessive disorder

    (D)   pain disorder

    (E)   masked depression

425. Longitudinal study has found that cryptic medical symptoms initially diagnosed as conversion disorder, pain disorder or hypochondriasis are sometimes early manifestations of any the following **EXCEPT**:

(A)   collagen vascular disease, e.g., lupus erythematosus
(B)   multiple sclerosis, myasthenia gravis
(C)   AIDS
(D)   essential hypertension
(E)   porphyria or other rare inborn error of metabolism

ANSWERS AND TUTORIAL ON ITEMS 418-425

The answers are: **418-E; 419-D; 420-D; 421-A; 422-E; 423-A, 424-B; 425-D**. The **somatoform disorders** section of DSM-IV attempts to classify various forms of aberrant illness behavior. The theoretical background mixes phenomenology, psychoanalytic ideas about defenses against directly dealing with conflict or stress, and common sense observations of patient behavior.

The term **somatization** comes from the psychoanalytic tradition and refers to the expression of emotion or distress in bodily rather than psychological terms. Like any other human psychological state, it reflects both aspects of the person and of the context in which it occurs. Personal factors include limited language capacity, which accounts for the commonness of somatization in young children. Other personal factors include those which explain why a person might want to be sick: desire to escape burdensome responsibilities or a desire to be taken care of by others.

Severe personal **traumas** may contribute to somatization, as shown by research findings that a substantial percentage of somaticizing patients have a history of traumatic experiences, especially child abuse. The explanation is that trauma, which by definition overwhelms normal ways of coping, arouses intense, distressing emotions which the patient suppresses but may experience as cryptic bodily sensations and express as illness. Traumas that violate deeply rooted beliefs about self and others or which occur when the person has very limited understanding of why such things might occur are particularly likely to distort normal emotional experience in this way. Children who are sexually or, to a lesser extent, physically abused, have difficulty communicating about their experience in words or handling the associated distress. Instead, they develop stomach aches, or dizziness, or pain, or some other bodily symptom. Somatization as a childhood behavior or as a commonly used defense in adults should prompt questions about previous traumatic experience.

While some people are probably innately disposed towards somatization, the behavior also seems to be learned and reinforced by various environmental and cultural factors. The early family environment of people who somatize is often one where someone in the family has a chronic illness, where parents are detached or distant but freely nurture a child who is ill, or where an important member somaticizes and is rewarded with attention and care. Children naturally gravitate toward behavior used by those they admire or identify with, especially if other ways of coping are not modelled or taught.

Culture also plays a role. Somatic expression of emotion is accepted and understood in many traditional cultures around the world. Although awareness of psychology is widespread in western culture, formal and informal discrimination against those with mental illness or psychological difficulties prompts some people to consciously or unconsciously magnify the bodily experience of emotion and disavow the cognitive aspects. The availability of technological medical resources is not known to be associated on either a personal or cultural level with somatization.

Frequent or significant resort to somatization as a defense is implied in many **somatoform disorders**, even though defensive somatization is not itself a diagnostic criterion. Descriptively, **conversion disorder**, one of Freud's original interests, is defined by the presence of a symptom or a few discreet symptoms that suggest a medical or neurological disease that cannot be confirmed. In psychoanalytic theory, conversion symptoms either symbolize or resolve an irresolvable conflict, as when a soldier cannot admit fear and instead experiences his arm as paralyzed in order to avoid return to battle. Contemporary understanding has broadened the concept of conversion to include symptoms that occur when a person is highly stressed, whether or not the stress reflects a conflict between conscious beliefs and postulated unconscious motives.

Other criteria require that the symptom cause significant impairment and not be solely pain or sexual dysfunction. Finally, diagnosis of conversion disorder requires that the person not consciously produce or feign the symptom--a difficult point to assess, but one that differentiates conversion disorder from factitious disorder and malingering (see below).

DSM-IV differentiates **pain disorder** from **conversion disorder**. The defining symptom of pain disorder is pain with no discoverable physical basis or which exceeds the normal distress associated with a particular illness. The pain, which cannot be sexual pain or a manifestation of another psychiatric disorder, is not consciously produced or feigned and must cause impairment.

As a diagnosis, pain disorder derives from the common sense experience of physicians who note that similar conditions produce enormous variations in distress. The psychological features of pain disorder include many of the elements of conversion disorder, that is, desire for the sick role, avoidance of internal or interpersonal conflict or overwhelming demand, bodily expression of inexpressible emotions, and rewards for illness behavior. The distinction between pain disorder and conversion disorder is more an artifact of the history of psychiatry than of valid differences in causality, but it is firmly embedded in current diagnostic schemes.

Psychoanalytic theory postulated a relationship between somaticizing and hysteria, a term that has fallen into disuse. **Histrionic personality disorder** incorporates some features of hysteria, specifically, seductiveness, dramatic emotional expression, and intense needs for attention. However, these qualities do not seem to be systematically or validly related to somatization, which occurs in people of many different personality types and disorders.

Somatization disorder is a diagnosis that comes from the descriptive phenomenological tradition. **Paul Briquet**, a French physician, provided an influential modern (1849) account of this condition, describing a syndrome of persistent, cryptic somatic complaints in multiple organ systems. The condition was called Briquet's syndrome until it was renamed somatization disorder in DSM-III (1977).

The **diagnostic criteria** for somatization disorder emphasize the number and distribution of symptoms (at least four pain symptoms, two gastrointestinal symptoms, one sexual symptom, and one pseudoneurological symptom), onset prior to age 30, impairment of function and absence of conscious feigning or illness production. Although most clinicians see somatization disorder as related to severe stress or conflict, this feature is not included in the diagnostic criteria. In any case, a single stress or traumatic event would be insufficient to cause the pervasive and long-standing symptoms required by the diagnosis.

As defined, the diagnosis is one of the most highly reliable in psychiatry. Epidemiological investigation has found the disorder in 0.5% of the general population. It has a 5:1 female to male predominance and may be found in up to 1% of women. There may be a genetic element: the concordance rate in monozygotic twins is twice that of dizygotic twins and an association exists between somatization disorder in women and substance abuse and antisocial personality disorder in men.

The presence of illness without verifiable evidence of a medical condition or disease is common both to the well-accepted psychiatric conditions of **conversion disorder**, **pain disorder**, and **somatization disorder**, and to **malingering**, a troubling and expensive behavior problem. A malingering person feigns or induces illness to escape some obligation or attain some concrete reward, such as legal damages or a pension. Physicians need to consider the possibility of a purposefully feigned illness when faced with patients who have inexplicable complaints or whose objective findings do not match their level of distress or impairment.

Whether symptoms are consciously or unconsciously produced is an important discrimination in current nosology. Conversion disorder is the correct answer in this item, because the description is of discreet symptoms not intentionally induced.

The other terms require definition. Malingering is described above. Patients with **factitious disorder** feign or even induce physical or psychological signs or symptoms. They may, for example, falsely claim to hallucinate or describe delusions, or use laxatives, diuretics, emetics, anticoagulants or insulin to produce objective manifestations of illness at some danger to themselves. Unlike malingerers, however, they are not seeking concrete rewards, such as pensions or legal damages. Rather, they seem to want to build or shore up their identity through being granted the sick role and receiving medical attention.

Munchausen's syndrome is a severe form of factitious disorder. Patients present with dramatic, feigned or induced alarming medical or psychiatric complaints and submit to all kinds of invasive treatment, including surgery, commitment to a hospital, or ECT.

Body dysmorphic disorder is an excessive preoccupation with some imagined or trivial physical defect (other than overweight), to the degree that interpersonal or occupational functioning is impaired. Although the condition results in avoidance of situations and demands for medical attention, it is not at all clear that these are the motivating factors. Body dysmorphic disorder may be a variant of obsessive-compulsive disorder, as it responds to similar treatment (SSRIs) 50% of the time.

The term **hypochondriasis** applies to excessive fears of having or developing a disease despite adequate medical reassurance. Hypochondriacal people often misinterpret bodily sensations as ominous, for example, they may think transient nausea means stomach cancer. Excessive worry or negative expectation is also a feature of anxiety disorders and depression. Hypochondriasis is diagnosed when the fears are confined to fears of disease and the other features of an anxiety or depressive disorder are absent. Malingering and pain disorder are defined above. Somatic obsessions is not a recognized term (see body dysmorphic disorder, above). "**Masked depression**" is also not an accepted term, although it has been used informally to describe people with some prominent symptom, like pain or hypochondriasis, who are found on systematic questioning to have many depressive symptoms which they have not mentioned spontaneously.

Longitudinal studies of patients diagnosed with **conversion disorder** have found that 40-60% have or later develop a diagnosable medical condition that may account for the cryptic symptoms. These conditions may be rare, have variable presentations, and be difficult to diagnose reliably. Essential hypertension is common and usually asymptomatic. Even if diagnosed in a patient with conversion disorder, it would not account for the symptoms which the patient displays. The point that patients with conversion disorder may be misdiagnosed does not render the diagnosis invalid, but should prompt physicians to make the diagnosis only after thoughtful screening. Medical evaluation should also occur if the symptoms do not respond to treatment or if new symptoms develop.

Select the **BEST** response.

426. Twenty-four hours after gallbladder surgery, a 30-year-old woman complains of pain and begs for a dose of meperidine 3 hours after receiving 50 mg IM. The **MOST** appropriate intervention would be

   (A)   Administer a saline placebo IM. Only accede to her request if she does not experience relief of her pain.
   (B)   Tell the patient that she needs to stick with the current regimen to avoid narcotic dependence and instruct the nursing staff to stick to the prescribed dosage schedule.
   (C)   Administer 75 mg and raise her standing dose to 75 mg every three hours if requested.
   (D)   Change her from meperidine to IV morphine, 5 mg push every four hours.

427. Three months after an episode of severe acute back pain, a 45-year-old man has chronic pain and requests a renewable prescription for propoxyphene, every three hours while awake, and a benzodiazepine for sleep. On physical examination, he has some tenderness and muscle spasm. Lifting his leg up straight brings on the pain. Medical evaluation including myelogram previously showed some degenerative joint disease of the spine, but no operable skeletai or disc pathology. His wife complains that he is "a big baby" and has her and the children waiting on him hand and foot. He is applying for disability, claiming his job as a warehouse manager, which included driving a forklift and some lifting, caused the problem. In addition to heat and physical therapy, the **MOST** appropriate intervention is

   (A)   Liberal administration of propoxyphene as requested, with laxatives to prevent constipation.
   (B)   Confrontation of his malingering and refusal to prescribe any further pain medication.
   (C)   Use of nonnarcotic analgesics and muscle relaxers, with the possible addition of an antidepressant. Family meetings to help the family have reasonable expectations for him to do as much for himself as he can.
   (D)   One week course of daily hypnosis, planting the suggestion he can make the pain go away at will; discontinuation of all pain medication.
   (E)   Discontinuation of all pain medication; termination from treatment and referral to an acupuncturist or chiropractor.

428. Self-controlled dosing of narcotics after surgery

   (A)   tends to result in better pain control
   (B)   does not typically prolong the time of narcotic use
   (C)   does not markedly increase the amount of narcotic taken
   (D)   A and C only
   (E)   A, B, and C

429. A positive response to the administration of a placebo for pain

   (A)   may be blocked by naltrexone
   (B)   is strongly suggestive of factitious disorder or malingering
   (C)   reliably predicts the person will respond to placebo the next time it is given
   (D)   A and C only
   (E)   A, B, and C

ANSWERS AND TUTORIAL ON ITEMS 426-429

The answers are: **426-C; 427-C; 428-E; 429-A.** The most common error in **treating acute pain** is underprescription of narcotics. **Meperidine**, in particular, is often given every four hours, but reliably wears off in three. Iatrogenic opiate addiction is extremely rare in patients taking narcotics for a clearcut medical indication. The use of a placebo is unethical if it is done to mislead a patient who has not consented to the possibility of receiving it. In any case, this patient's response to a placebo would be of no diagnostic value. Pain from any cause is always subjective and modified by personal and environmental variables. Manipulation of these variables by giving a placebo does not prove the pain has no "real" basis.

Since anxious anticipation tends to worsen pain, many hospitals now allow patients to regulate their own dose of narcotic analgesics, using an IV system that delivers a bolus of medication when a button is pressed. This method relieves patients' anxiety that the pain will return as soon as the current dose wears off or if the next dose is delayed. In general, because patients do not experience as much pain, they tend to use less opiates. Weaning is no harder than for patients treated with caregiver controlled methods. The one disadvantage is that the IV dosage route may speed up the development of tolerance.

The therapeutic strategy for **chronic pain** differs from that for acute pain. Indeed, the two conditions may be neurologically different, with the fibers capable of sustained transmission of pain sensation being less responsive to opiates than those that subserve acute pain. Even though this patient is applying for disability, it would be inappropriate to assume he is malingering; he has objective findings supporting his complaint, and his work conditions, in fact, could have contributed to his problem. Pending legal proceedings do seem to impede full rehabilitation and recovery, but malingering is not necessarily the reason. All symptoms, but especially pain, are affected by how much attention a patient pays to them. Patients naturally focus on their distress while engaged in the lengthy, and sometimes humiliating and adversarial process of trying to prove the validity of their complaints.

Free use of an opiate-like drug, however, is not an effective treatment for chronic pain. Patients tend, over time, to become tolerant to the analgesic effect of opiates, while also developing physiological dependence.

Some degree of inflammation may contribute to pain even from obvious anatomical lesions, and nonnarcotic, anti-inflammatory agents may be effective. This patient's muscle spasms may also be contributing to his pain. Antidepressants have been shown to improve chronic pain in some people, whether or not the person is depressed.

Pain is also a form of communication. Teaching family members to be less attentive to the patients' complaints and more appreciative or encouraging of the ways they continue to function can reduce expressions of pain and demands for relief, presumably actually helping the person to feel less distress.

Hypnosis is useful in the treatment of chronic pain. However, it is not administered intensively for a brief period, as described. Patients are taught to hypnotize themselves and to transform the pain sensations into something else. They also learn to relax by imagining themselves into serene, safe settings. They must be motivated to practice self-hypnosis on a regular basis for the treatment to be effective. Teaching people the technique may take only a single session; others may require booster sessions spread over more than one week.

Acupuncture may be an effective intervention for chronic pain, but it is not rigorously proven. In any case, referral to an acupuncturist or a chiropractor should not involve rejecting the patient for further medical treatment. Both methods succeed in part due to practitioners' skill in establishing a strong therapeutic alliance with a patient, providing a convincing explanation of how treatment works, and engaging the patient in rituals that symbolize healing. Acupuncture, in addition, may work by stimulating pain fibers proximal to the area of pathology, so that distal stimuli are blocked (gating). Chiropractic relieves muscle spasms with various kinds of manipulation. A mainstream practitioner can mobilize many of the same therapeutic elements, if he or she is caring, competent and nonjudgmental and knows how to use nondrug rehabilitation methods, including exercise, massage, heat, and hypnosis.

The **placebo response** is not fully understood. As noted above, it does not reliably differentiate real from feigned illness; patients with obvious, severe pathology may respond. It is also highly unpredictable--the same patient may respond on one occasion and not on another, under identical circumstances. No particular personality type responds or does not respond. One intriguing finding is that naltrexone, an opiate receptor blocker, may prevent the placebo response, indicating that it may be mediated by the release of endogenous opiates.

Items 430-437

A 25-year-old college student who is of normal weight seeks treatment from the counselling center for depression, fatigue, and feelings of self-loathing. She gives a history of significant fluctuations in weight since adolescence, never dropping below the lowest normal weight for height or becoming amenorrheic. She is preoccupied with weight and calorie counting, restricts her social life to avoid situations where she might be tempted to overeat, and admits to using laxatives to keep her weight down after she has "cheated" on her diet. A "cheating" episode may involve secretly eating a pint of ice cream or having two dinners in a row.

430.   Her diagnosis is **MOST** likely

    (A)   bulimia nervosa
    (B)   atypical depression
    (C)   anorexia nervosa
    (D)   body dysmorphic disorder
    (E)   None of the above

431.   Patients with this disorder

    (A)   Have diminished self-worth and equate their value with their physical appearance.
    (B)   Will have comorbid anxiety or depression or substance abuse up to 75% of the time.
    (C)   May become socially isolated in order to conceal their eating behavior.
    (D)   A and C only
    (E)   A, B, and C

432.   Appropriate treatment may include

    (A)   nutritional counselling and education about the effects and dangers of her eating habits
    (B)   group therapy with other young women with similar problems
    (C)   a serotonin-specific reuptake inhibitor
    (D)   A and C only
    (E)   A, B, and C

A sixteen-year-old girl who was 5'3" and weighed 145 lbs at her last pediatric visit comes in for evaluation of amenorrhea. She now weighs 100 lbs. She reports that she lost weight through completely eliminating all fatty foods, limiting carbohydrates, and running five miles per day. She expresses the wish to loose another ten pounds. On questioning, she admits to feeling cold easily but denies that she is tired or hungry. She goes into great detail about each thing that she eats, and she becomes angry when the physician suggests she is underweight.

433. Her diagnosis is **MOST** likely

    (A)   bulimia nervosa
    (B)   Sheehan's syndrome
    (C)   anorexia nervosa
    (D)   adjustment disorder with mixed disturbance of emotions and conduct
    (E)   body dysmorphic disorder

434. Without treatment, the lifetime mortality associated with her condition is

    (A)   insignificant
    (B)   1-7%
    (C)   5-18%
    (D)   15-20%
    (E)   greater than 20%

435. Her condition occurs

    (A)   in 0.5-1% of all women
    (B)   10-20X more frequently in women than in men
    (C)   more in industrialized than nonindustrialized societies
    (D)   A and C only
    (E)   A, B, and C

436. The salient psychological concerns found in this disorder include all **EXCEPT**:

    (A)   discomfort with mature female sexuality
    (B)   deficient sense of autonomy or efficacy; compensatory efforts to feel powerful by controlling eating and body size
    (C)   excessive desires for specialness, perfectionism
    (D)   cognitive distortions, such as overgeneralization, all-or-nothing thinking, and catastrophic thinking, mainly focussed around eating
    (E)   anxiety over the health consequences of being underweight

437. Initial treatment may include

   (A) Involving her parents in behavioral contracting, with privileges such as being allowed to exercise or attend school or spend time with friends being strictly tied to gradual increase in weight.
   (B) Immediate initiation of psychodynamic psychotherapy to explore her fears of sexuality and other developmental issues and conflicts.
   (C) Treatment with a tricyclic or monoamine oxidase inhibiting antidepressant.
   (D) A and C only
   (E) A, B, and C

ANSWERS AND TUTORIAL ON ITEMS 430-437

The answers are: **430-A; 431-D; 432-E; 433-C; 434-C; 435-E; 436-E; 437-A**. The 25-year-old college student has **bulimia nervosa**. Anorexia nervosa requires that the person refuse to maintain a weight over 85% of normal and be amenorrheic. Many anorexics do become bulimic later on. In DSM-IV, prior diagnosis of anorexia precludes the diagnosis of bulimia; such a patient would be given the diagnosis of "anorexia nervosa: binge eating/purging type." Although patients with either anorexia nervosa or bulimia nervosa may have gross distortions of body image, by definition, body dysmorphic disorder excludes preoccupation with weight and thinness. Major depression with atypical features connotes depression with hypersomnia, hyperphagia, and preserved capacity for pleasure. While the condition may occur along with bulimia nervosa, it does not captures the primary symptoms of binging and purging, which require the diagnosis of bulimia nervosa.

Bulimia nervosa responds well to a variety of treatments. Patients first need to regain control of their uncontrolled behavior. A balanced diet of small frequent meals will help relieve the intense hunger that provokes the binges, which the patient purges to reverse. Patients often have idiosyncratic ideas about food and eat unbalanced diets as a way of losing weight. Thus, nutritional counselling is an important part of the treatment.

The immediate focus of group therapy is educating patients about how starvation produces food preoccupations, binging, and feelings of fatigue and loss of control. Once they are less symptomatic, many patients with this disorder become aware of the psychological distress that they were managing by focussing on eating/not eating or purging. A therapy group with other sufferers can relieve shame and self-loathing and promote a healthy sense of personal value that does not depend on body shape. Finally, serotonin-specific reuptake inhibitors, monamine oxidase inhibitors, and tricyclic antidepressants have all proven helpful to more severely ill patients. These drugs are effective whether or not the person is concurrently depressed. They seem to help patients feel satiated after eating, quickly reducing the number and extent of their binges.

The 16-year-old girl is presenting the typical picture of **anorexia nervosa**: refusal to maintain a weight 85% of normal, amenorrhea, preoccupation with food, and lack of insight into the distortions of thinking that support the desire to be so thin. The relationship between bulimia nervosa and anorexia nervosa is detailed above; this patient has the "restricting type" of her disease. Body dysmorphic disorder, also described above, specifically excludes misperceptions of body size. Sheehan's syndrome (panhypopituitarism due to pituitary hemorrhage) shares with anorexia nervosa the development of cold intolerance, amenorrhea, and sometimes weakness or cachexia. However, it typically occurs as a complication of pregnancy, and the desire to be thin is not a prominent feature. Adjustment disorder requires the presence of an event or circumstance that triggers a patient's symptoms. No such event is described here.

Anorexia nervosa is a serious, relatively common disorder (0.5-1% of women) with a significant mortality rate--5-18%. It is 10-20 times more frequent in females than males, although the number of men diagnosed with this disorder is increasing. It may be found in every ethnic group or social class, but it is quite uncommon in nonindustrial societies. Bulimia nervosa is more common--1-2% of women in the U.S. - but its mortality rate is not high enough to report.

Patients with anorexia nervosa are less generally impulsive than those with bulimia nervosa. The disease puts them at odds with their families, who can become frantic over patients' refusal to eat normally. This has led many observers to postulate that a desire to establish autonomy, implying a pre-existing problem with separation and independence, may motivate or sustain the disorder. Patients are also highly responsive to messages in the culture about the glamour of being thin, indicating a need to be perfect and special. While these patients are able to exercise an extraordinary degree of control over their eating, they often seem to be overcompensating for feelings of confusion, inefficacy, and incompetence in other areas. They are characteristically *unconcerned* with the effects of being so underweight.

The **treatment of anorexia nervosa**, like that of bulimia nervosa, must begin with reversing the state of semi-starvation. Otherwise, the patient remains preoccupied with food and control of eating, and nothing else engages her. Bulimics are often motivated to stop their maladaptive behavior. Anorexics are typically far more resistant. A degree of coercion is often necessary at the outset. For younger, less sick patients, the family can learn to tie desired rewards, such as privacy, or permission to exercise, or greater independence, to specific amounts of regained weight. Sicker patients will require hospitalization. Even if they are admitted voluntarily, they often struggle desperately against whatever measures are taken to get them to regain weight.

Once in nutritional balance, but not until then, anorexic patients may undergo psychodynamic therapy, usually on an individual basis. The sense of inefficacy and confusion that go along with anorexia nervosa make group treatment with these patients rather more difficult than with bulimics, who tend to be more mature, with a wider range of normal coping behaviors. Antidepressants have not proven generally effective for patients with anorexia nervosa, though there are case reports of responses to particular agents.

Items 438-442

Match the personality disorder in the list with the **MOST** typical defining qualities in the items below. Answers may be used once, more than once, or not at all.

- (A)   Avoidant
- (B)   Dependent
- (C)   Obsessive-compulsive
- (D)   Schizoid
- (E)   Schizotypal
- (F)   Antisocial
- (G)   Histrionic
- (H)   Narcissistic
- (I)   Borderline
- (J)   Paranoid

438.   Self-important, grandiose, lacking in empathy, envious; feels entitled to special consideration, respect.

439.   Peculiar thinking with nondelusional ideas of reference; inappropriate/constricted affect; odd, eccentric behavior and speech; illusions; lack of close friends except first degree relatives; excessive, inextinguishable social anxiety.

440.   Wants to be the center of attention; seductive or provocative interpersonally; self-dramatizing; rapidly shifting, shallow emotion; impressionistic cognitive style.

441.   Desires relationships but does not pursue them for fear of shame or ridicule; limits occupational choices for fear of criticism, disapproval or rejection; feelings of being inept, inferior, inadequate.

442.   Lacks desire for close relationships, even with family; lacking in sexual interest; emotionally detached, flattened affect; strongly prefers solitary activities.

Choose the **BEST** response.

A physician is treating a 60-year-old immigrant man for emphysema. He notes the patient is mistrustful and uncooperative. The patient believes the cause of his disease was exposure to air-born pollutants at an industrialized farm he worked on 30 years ago, prior to his immigration. He resents and discounts any counsel that his heavy smoking might be a contributory factor. He changes doctors frequently, claiming that various previous treating physicians were incompetent, discriminating against him because he is foreign born, or trying to keep him sick to increase their income. However, he is sure that his present doctor will be different, knowing him to be the "best". He is divorced after a marriage during which he admits to having several affairs. He describes his ex-wife as exploitative and untrustworthy, mentioning that he knew she was also unfaithful, with no concrete proof except "the way she started looking at other men."

443.   This presentation would be **MOST** consistent with a diagnosis of

      (A)   schizoid personality disorder
      (B)   paranoid personality disorder
      (C)   borderline personality disorder
      (D)   schizotypal personality disorder
      (E)   antisocial personality disorder

Upon further questioning, the patient describes his early life as happy, with good family relationships and close friends. During a guerilla war in his home country, many of these friends were killed or disappeared; he suspects that one of them may have betrayed his brother, who was then shot. He came to the US illegally at age 35 and lived in constant fear of being sent home until successfully applying for asylum. During the years he lacked legal status, he was unable to get competent medical care, and he could not get compensation when a truck in the warehouse where he worked ran over his foot. He describes a few current friends, mostly fellow refugees who have similar experiences and attitudes.

444.   This further history suggests that the diagnosis of a personality disorder, as defined in DSM-IV, is not justified because

      (A)   The patient's dysfunctional attitudes were not clearly present until middle adulthood.
      (B)   The patient's dysfunctional attitudes are understandable in light of his earlier experience.
      (C)   There is evidence, based on his friendships, that the patient's attitudes are not far off those of others in his cultural group.
      (D)   A and C only
      (E)   A, B, and C only

445. The psychological defenses shown by this patient include

   (A) projection
   (B) dissociation
   (C) splitting
   (D) A and C only
   (E) A, B, and C only

During a major depressive episode, a 32-year-old woman becomes anxious and distressed whenever she is alone in her house. She is obviously overqualified for her job, but avoids looking for a better one because she feels she couldn't handle working with people she doesn't already know. She works long hours so as to avoid being home in the evenings. She has a boyfriend she describes as "kind of a loser," but she stays with him in order not to be alone. During the course of her initial interview, she asks the primary care clinician whether she should look for another job and dump this boyfriend.

446. Although a number of personality disorders may be present, this picture is most consistent with

   (A) avoidant personality disorder
   (B) borderline personality disorder
   (C) dependent personality disorder
   (D) histrionic personality disorder
   (E) obsessive-compulsive personality disorder

447. To confirm this woman's diagnosis of personality disorder according to DSM-IV criteria, the evaluator must establish that

   (A) The patient has difficulty making decisions, being alone, and accepting challenges during periods of her life when she is not depressed.
   (B) The patient was never a victim of child abuse or any traumatic experience that might have induced her current attitudes.
   (C) Similar personality traits have been found in some of her first or second degree relatives.
   (D) A and C only
   (E) A, B, and C

448. By definition, the DSM-IV personality disorders

   (A) Exist in people with no discernible biological abnormality.
   (B) May be understood as arrest at immature stages of development.
   (C) Constitute a clear indication for psychodynamic psychotherapy.
   (D) All of the above.
   (E) None of the above.

ANSWERS AND TUTORIAL ON ITEMS 438-448

The answers are: **438-H; 439-E; 440-G; 441-A; 442-D; 443-B; 444-D; 445-D; 446-C; 447-A; 448-E.** The concept of **personality disorder** connotes persistent and pervasive problems of adaptation, manifested in mood, thinking, self-concept, and patterns of relating to others. The DSM-IV defines personality disorder very stringently. The main criteria for five personality disorders are given above. The presence of one or two of these criteria would be considered personality **traits**. The diagnosis of personality disorder requires that patients exhibit a specified range of maladaptive qualities over many years, beginning at the latest by early adulthood. The traits must also influence behavior in several different contexts. The diagnosis of personality disorder is excluded if the pattern observed seems to reflect subcultural variation. Dependent traits and behaviors, for example, are reinforced, even instilled, in women in many cultures around the world. A woman whose culture teaches her to rely heavily on others and limit her choices based on others' opinions or fears of abandonment would not merit the diagnosis of dependent personality disorder. Someone with the same traits might warrant the diagnosis if she were raised in a culture that stressed independence and autonomy.

Because of the exclusion criteria, a personality disorder diagnosis cannot be given the 60-year-old patient above. He does have pervasive, persistent difficulties manifested in several contexts. His mistrust, for example, affected both his marriage in the past and his current ability to use medical care. However, his difficulties seem to have begun later than early adulthood and may reflect the values and attitudes of a minority culture. Whether or not a person's problems are understandable--that is, how they reflect either unique life experience or derive from some theoretical model of development--is irrelevant in making DSM-IV diagnoses, though clinically of great importance.

Although he does not qualify for a DSM-IV diagnosis, current theories of personality development and functioning do contribute to the categorization of this man's difficulties. His mistrust, while understandable in the context of his life experience and not clearly at variance with reality, is nevertheless excessive and maladaptive. By mistrusting doctors who confront his smoking, for example, he compromises his health. His seeing infidelity in his wife without acknowledging it in himself suggests that he uses the defense of projection (see chapter II), perceiving his own inner experience as coming from outside the self. His global statements that all doctors are bad, yet his current doctor is the best suggest that he also uses splitting. That is, he experiences others dichotomously as all good/all bad, completely indifferent/unstintingly caring, etc. This way of relating suggests that when he is ambivalent towards another person, he suppresses one or the other arm of his ambivalence as a way of maintaining a coherent world-view. Mistrust, projection, and the attribution of malevolence are all elements of paranoia, which may be either psychotic, implying a break from reality, or nonpsychotic, as in personality disorder. Splitting, while not automatically linked to paranoia, is an immature defense similar to projection. The two often co-occur.

The other terms in the list, **schizoid, borderline, schizotypal** and **antisocial**, all have specific definitions. **Schizoid** describes people who are uninterested in social attachment. Schizotypal people have both diminished capacity for relationships and peculiar patterns of thought, including magical thinking, odd beliefs, odd perceptual experiences, and subtle, low grade abnormalities of thought form. Borderline traits include impulsivity, unstable relationships driven by fears of abandonment, problems of identity, chronic feelings of emptiness, suicidal thinking and behavior, and dysphoric moods, including irritability. Antisociality describes disregard for the rights of others shown in lack of remorse. People with this disorder also show irritability and aggressiveness, risk taking, irresponsibility and impulsivity.

As described, this patient's most prominent personality abnormalities are nonpsychotically distorted thinking and social alienation/mistrust. Were it not for the exclusion criteria outlined above, his behavior would be consistent with the diagnosis of paranoid personality disorder.

The 32-year-old woman is demonstrating **dependent traits**: indecisiveness, intolerance of being alone, lack of self-confidence, and going to excessive lengths to obtain nurturance and support from others. Her asking the doctor for personal (not medical) advice at a first meeting, for example, suggests she seeks reassurance from others rather than relying on her own judgment. Staying in an unsatisfactory relationship to avoid being alone is a core feature of maladaptive dependency.

As described, this patient does not present the qualities of **avoidant personality**. That is, she does not wish for relationships but fail to pursue them out of fears of rejection, criticism or ridicule. While one may infer she has low self-esteem, which is an aspect of avoidant personality, she makes her choices out of fears of feeling isolated, rather than because of self-doubt or the expectation of being disliked. **Histrionic personality** connotes people who are dramatic, seductive, suggestible and shallow. Efforts have been made to define histrionicity in gender blind terms, though it derives from the earlier concept of hysterical personality that applied mainly to women. That this patient seeks advice inappropriately might be seen as seductive, but the other qualities of histrionicity are not described. The impulsivity, extreme emotion and self-destructiveness of **borderline personality** are not evident in this case, although fear of abandonment is a trait shared with dependent personality disorder. **Obsessive-compulsive personality** describes people who are perfectionistic, preoccupied with rules and order, overconscientious, rigid, stubborn and stingy. Like this patient, many obsessive-compulsive people work excessive hours and for idiosyncratic reasons that do not reflect economic necessity or the real demands of their jobs. Again, the presence of this disorder is not ruled out by the description given, but it is not the most probable diagnosis.

It is important to stress that many of the major syndromes are associated with abnormal moods, perceptions, interpersonal behaviors and subjective beliefs. In order to diagnose personality disorders, these qualities must persist at times when the person is not in the middle of an illness that might cause them. Depression, in particular, seems to accentuate dependent and avoidant traits, which may become clinically insignificant when the depression remits. Appearance of these traits during a depressive episode does not warrant a personality disorder diagnosis.

Except for making culture an exclusion criterion, DSM-IV avoids linking personality dysfunction to the presence or absence of prior experience that might have contributed to it. While it may be very important in treatment planning to know if this patient's early experience was traumatic and not conducive to the development of an independent, mature self-concept, such understanding does not contribute to her diagnosis. Similarly, although some of the personality disorders appear to reflect inherited characteristics, the presence or absence of a family history is not a core diagnostic criterion.

The original formulations of personality in psychiatry emphasized uneven development or developmental arrest, but these formulations are not explicit in the phenomenologically defined personality disorders. Moreover, although people with personality disorders need not have a definable physiological abnormality, it is not true that personality disorders, as currently defined, are unrelated to biology. Various abnormal qualities of personality--anxiety in the face of minor disruptions of attachment, impulsivity, lack of emotion, and peculiar thinking--have all been studied as manifestations of neurological processes. Indeed, the fact that some of the personality disorders, especially antisocial, avoidant, and schizotypal personality, have significant familial incidence or are linked to disorders with significant genetic loading suggests that biological mechanisms play an important role. For this reason, among others, the diagnosis of a personality disorder does not immediately indicate that psychotherapy is the appropriate treatment. Psychotherapists have traditionally studied and treated personality disorders, but recognition of possible neurologic mechanisms contributing to maladaptive traits are opening the way to pharmacologic treatments for some aspects of these disorders.

Moreover, personality disorders are, by definition, **ego-syntonic** (the person does not see his/her traits as different from normal self). They are typically recognized incidentally, when people seek care because their adaptation has broken down--they become distressed after a relationship ends or they lose a job or they cannot cope with a medical illness. Psychodynamic psychotherapy is only appropriate for patients who demonstrate some capacity for insight and are motivated to change. It would be indicated in personality disordered patients who recognize that they have precipitated or contributed to their own maladaptation. Behavioral and supportive psychotherapies, by design, do not focus on trying to change the person's sense of self. They may help patients with personality disorders who would not likely benefit from psychodynamic psychotherapy.

<u>Items</u> <u>449-453</u>

Match the personality disorder on the list to the major syndrome in the items with which it is associated. Answers may be used once, more than once, or not at all.

(A) Avoidant
(B) Schizotypal
(C) Borderline
(D) Antisocial
(E) Narcissistic
(F) Histrionic
(G) Paranoid

449. Schizophrenia

450. Somatization disorder

451. Social phobia

452. Posttraumatic stress disorder (PTSD)

453. Hypomania

ANSWERS AND TUTORIAL ON ITEMS 449-453

The answers are: **449-B; 450-D; 451-A; 452-C; 453-E.** Different conditions diagnosed on axis I relate to some of the personality disorders through genetics, shared symptoms, or shared causal mechanisms. Many people have noted that certain forms of schizophrenia, especially undifferentiated and disorganized subtypes, rarely occur in people with previously normal personalities. Genetic research has linked **schizotypal personality disorder** to schizophrenia, raising the possibility that people with some genetic loading for schizophrenia may demonstrate schizotypal personality disorder without developing the full-blown disorder. Patients with schizotypal personality disorder may also be in the premorbid phase of schizophrenia. The relationship between schizoid personality and schizophrenia is far less clear.

Although phenomenologically quite different, **somatization disorder** and **antisocial personality disorder** are linked in genetic studies showing significantly increased rates of antisocial personality and substance abuse in the close male relatives of women with somatization disorder. Histrionic personality is not systematically linked to somatization. This is a significant negative finding refuting past theories that linked conversion symptoms and somatization to hysteria, the earlier formulation of histrionic personality.

As currently defined, **avoidant personality disorder** and social phobia, generalized type, overlap to a large extent. The diagnoses are not mutually exclusive. Patients with avoidant personality disorder may develop social phobia or meet criteria concurrently for both disorders. The main difference is that people with avoidant personality disorder need not describe acute anxiety attacks in social situations as the cause of their social inhibition.

Many theorists now link **borderline personality disorder** to early traumatic experience, especially sexual abuse. While not expressed in the diagnostic criteria, some borderline patients will, if asked, report traumatic experiences and such symptoms as intrusive recollection, flashbacks, physiological distress when reminded, irritability, and hopelessness. These are defining criteria of PTSD. Conversely, adults who experience catastrophic repetitive trauma may exhibit borderline qualities in unstable relationships that alternate between clinging and detachment, rage, unstable affect, emptiness, impulsivity and suicidality. Although the early onset criterion of DSM-IV excludes such patients from receiving a borderline personality diagnosis, the International Classification of Diseases (ICD)-10 does include a code for enduring personality change after catastrophic experience, defined in terms that mirror the definition of borderline personality disorder in the DSM-IV.

The psychological features of **hypomania** resemble those of **narcissistic personality** to a large extent. Hypomanic patients have a grandiose sense of self that may lead to expectations of recognition or special treatment from others. Arrogance, fantasies of success or ideal love, and exploitation of others, all criteria of narcissistic personality, may also occur in someone who is hypomanic. People who experience frequent or prolonged upswings of mood may demonstrate these qualities even when they are not clearly in a state different from normal or demonstrating neurovegetative signs. The overlap of the two disorders may reflect shared genetic factors or mechanisms or result from the effect of chronic mental illness upon personality. A category for personality change or deterioration after persistent mental illness exists in the ICD-10 but not in DSM-IV.

CHAPTER X
SLEEP AND SLEEP DISORDERS

Items 454-460

Sleep EEG (polysomnographic) tracings are shown in **Figure 10.1** below.

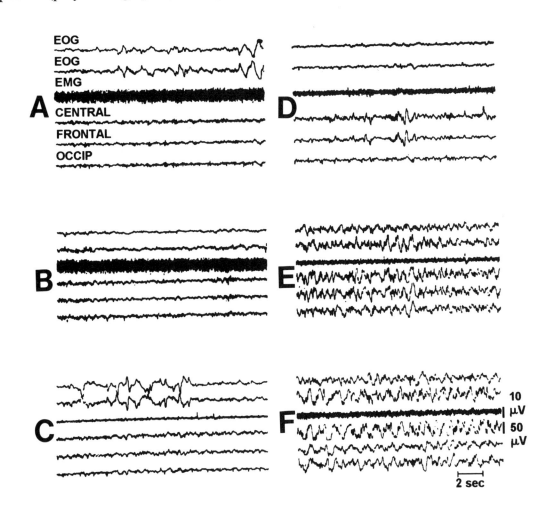

Figure 10.1

Choose the **BEST** response.

454.   Which tracing was recorded during REM sleep?

(A)   A
(B)   B
(C)   C
(D)   D
(E)   E
(F)   F

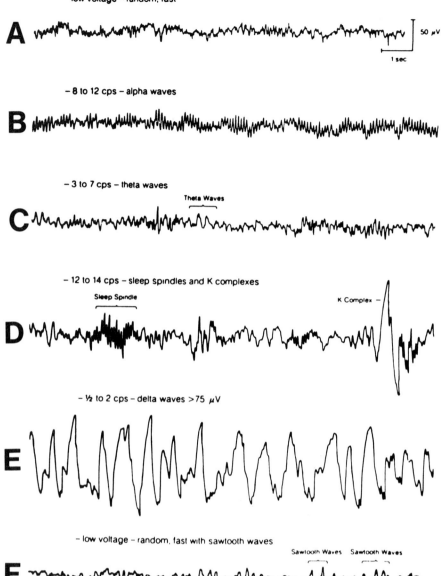

Figure 10.2

455. Which of the above EEG lead tracings shown in **Figure 10.2** above is characteristic of stage 2 sleep?

    (A)   A
    (B)   B
    (C)   C
    (D)   D
    (E)   E
    (F)   F

Choose the **BEST** response.

456. During the first ninety minutes of sleep

    (A) Normal people go through four distinct EEG stages.
    (B) Normal sleep stages alternate with microawakenings (stage 0) that subside during the rest of the night.
    (C) Normal people experience the first two rapid eye movement (REM) periods of the night.
    (D) A and C only
    (E) A, B, and C

457. The regulation of REM sleep is principally

    (A) noradrenergic
    (B) cholinergic
    (C) serotonergic
    (D) dopaminergic
    (E) None of the above

458. REM sleep

    (A) corresponds with dreaming
    (B) normally occupies 25% of total sleep time in adults
    (C) occurs mostly in the last third of the night
    (D) A and C only
    (E) A, B, and C

459. Delta or slow wave sleep (stage 3-4)

    (A) normally occupies 25% of total sleep time in adults
    (B) increases with old age
    (C) is associated with no mental activity and the highest arousal threshold
    (D) A and C only
    (E) A, B, and C

460. The regulation of nonrapid eye movement (NREM) sleep is principally

    (A) noradrenergic
    (B) cholinergic
    (C) serotonergic
    (D) dopaminergic
    (E) None of the above

ANSWERS AND TUTORIAL ON ITEMS 454-460

The answers are: **454-C; 455-D; 456-A; 457-A; 458-E; 459-D; 460-C**. An orderly progression of patterned brain activity occurs in cycles throughout **normal sleep** in human beings. This progression, called **sleep architecture**, goes from **wakefulness** (Stage 0) to **drowsiness** (Stage 1), **sleep onset** (Stage 2-appearance of sleep spindles and K complexes on EEG), **deep sleep** or **delta sleep** correlates with (Stages 3 and 4--high voltage delta waves on EEG) and **rapid eye movement sleep** (REM). Brain activity during REM sleep closely resembles wakefulness (random fast activity or 8-12 cps, low voltage alpha waves with intermixed beta 13-35 cps waves) with eyes closed, but with two important differences: rapid conjugate eye movements and total muscular paralysis.

In Items 454-455, answer C, in **Figure 10.1**, which shows the eye movements on lines one and two and the lack of muscle movement on line 3, is a depiction of **REM sleep**. (A is stage 1, B is stage 2, C is stage 4). Tracing D, in **Figure 10.2**, illustrates **sleep spindles** and **K complexes**, characteristic of **stage 2**.

Normal sleep architecture involves progression from stage 2-4 and back again, with periods of REM following stage 2 and occurring in place of stage 1 or 0. That is, people go into periods of deep (stage 3-4) sleep, approach wakefulness, enter REM, and then return to deep sleep. The REM periods lengthen in the latter third of the night and stage 3 and 4 gradually diminish. Both REM and deep sleep periods occupy 25% of total sleep time. The first sleep cycle of the night typically lasts ninety minutes and includes the longest period of deep or delta sleep. Neither REM nor brief awakening time typically occur during this phase of sleep.

The physiology of sleep is still obscure, but **serotonin** appears to regulate NREM sleep and **norepinephrine** seems to be the primary regulator of REM sleep. Acetylcholine is involved in maintaining the normal progression of sleep stages. These findings come from selective ablation studies, in which destruction or inhibition of serotonin-containing **raphe nuclei** leads to total insomnia, destruction or inhibition of the noradrenergic **locus ceruleus** neurons abolishes REM sleep, and loss of cholinergic function in **dementia** correlates with fragmentation of sleep. Dopamine is not implicated in the regulation of sleep in current physiologic models.

It is useful to contrast **REM sleep** and **deep sleep**, the poles of the normal sleep cycle. Each occupies 25% of total sleep time. Deep sleep predominates in the first third of the night and may not occur at all in the last third. REM begins after the first ninety minutes of sleep and increases to its highest percentage as stage 3-4 disappears. People awakened during REM sleep typically report dreams. Those awakened from stage three or four report no ideation. The arousal threshold rises from stage 1 to stage 4. Patients in deep sleep are the most difficult to awaken. The arousal threshold during REM varies. Patients in REM sleep are close to awakening by all physiological parameters except muscle tone. Deep sleep and REM sleep both **decrease** in old age, though REM sleep never disappears entirely. The absence of deep sleep in old age correlates with complaints of nonrestful sleep and daytime drowsiness in elderly people.

Choose the **BEST** response.

461. In general population surveys

    (A)   up to 35% of adults report sleep problems
    (B)   sleep problems rise with rising socioeconomic status
    (C)   sleep problems are reported as serious in 17% of adults
    (D)   A and C only
    (E)   A, B, and C

462. Inadequate sleep is associated with

    (A)   decreased work efficiency and productivity
    (B)   traffic accidents
    (C)   increased rates of cardiovascular disease
    (D)   A and C only
    (E)   A, B, and C

463. After a period of sleep deprivation, which phases will rebound (be more prolonged or intense) at the expense of other sleep stages?

    (A)   delta sleep only
    (B)   REM sleep only
    (C)   stages 1-2, REM
    (D)   delta sleep and REM sleep
    (E)   None. Total sleep will increase with roughly the same proportion of stages as sleep prior to the sleep deprivation.

464. DSM-IV categorizes all of the following as dyssomnias **EXCEPT**:

    (A)   difficulty initiating or maintaining sleep (insomnia)
    (B)   excessive daytime sleepiness (hypersomnia)
    (C)   breathing-related sleep abnormalities (sleep apnea)
    (D)   sleepwalking (somnambulism)
    (E)   circadian rhythm sleep disorder

465. Patients with primary insomnia without sleep apnea, narcolepsy, or underlying psychiatric disorder should be instructed to

    (A)   go to bed at the same time every night
    (B)   get out of bed at the same time every morning
    (C)   read or watch TV in bed until they fall asleep
    (D)   A and C only
    (E)   A, B, and C

466. Narcolepsy

    (A)   is characterized by sudden onset of sleep during either monotonous or normal waking activity

    (B)   is associated with markedly increased REM latency (time to the onset of REM sleep) on sleep EEG

    (C)   is associated with a positive family history (narcolepsy in a first degree relative) less than 10% of the time

    (D)   A and C only

    (E)   A, B, and C

467. The **MOST** common auxiliary symptom in narcolepsy is

    (A)   hypnagogic hallucinations

    (B)   sleep paralysis

    (C)   cataplexy

    (D)   snoring

    (E)   enuresis

468. Sleep apnea is associated with all the following **EXCEPT**:

    (A)   loud snoring

    (B)   morning headaches

    (C)   enuresis

    (D)   nocturnal gastroesophageal reflux

    (E)   orthostatic hypotension

469. On polysomnography, sleep apnea appears as

    (A)   frequent microawakenings

    (B)   multiple periods of cessation of respiration lasting 10 seconds or more

    (C)   decreased stage 3/4 sleep

    (D)   A and C only

    (E)   A, B, and C

470. The difference between central and obstructive sleep apnea is that

    (A)   Patients with obstructive apnea have increased thoracic over diaphragmatic respiratory effort during episodes.

    (B)   Patients with central apnea fail to show respiratory effort during apneic episodes.

    (C)   Patients with central apnea have longer and more frequent episodes.

    (D)   Patients with obstructive apnea more commonly awaken with headaches from muscle tension.

471. Sleep apnea

    (A)   has a 10:1 male:female ratio in incidence prior to menopause
    (B)   rises drastically in prevalence in old age
    (C)   causes significant impairment in relationships (60+%), occupational functioning (80+%), and general health
    (D)   A and C only
    (E)   A, B, and C

472. Findings or conditions associated with sleep apnea include all the following **EXCEPT**:

    (A)   hypoglycemia
    (B)   obesity
    (C)   hypertension
    (D)   allergies or chronic sinus obstruction
    (E)   hypothyroidism

473. Sleep apnea

    (A)   may lead to significant psychosocial dysfunction
    (B)   impairs sexual function in some patients
    (C)   leads to increased mortality if persistent and untreated
    (D)   All of the above
    (E)   None of the above

474. A 25-year-old medical student complains that he cannot get to sleep before 4 AM then sleeps seven hours, frequently missing morning classes. This case exemplifies

    (A)   advanced sleep phase syndrome
    (B)   REM sleep behavior disorder
    (C)   delayed sleep phase syndrome
    (D)   psychophysiologic insomnia
    (E)   adjustment sleep disorder

475. The difference between nocturnal myoclonus and restless legs syndrome is that

    (A)   patients are unaware of any limb sensations with nocturnal myoclonus
    (B)   patients with myoclonus complain of frequent awakenings; patients with restless legs have difficulty falling asleep
    (C)   myoclonus is found in association with sleep apnea and narcolepsy; restless legs is associated more with mood disorders and psychosocial distress
    (D)   A and C only
    (E)   A, B, and C

The answers are: **461-D; 462-E; 463-D; 464-D; 465-B; 466-A; 467-C; 468-E; 469-E; 470-B; 471-E; 472-A; 473-D; 474-C; 475-E. Insomnia** is a common complaint, experienced by roughly 35% of people at some time in the past year in general population surveys. Half this number, 17%, have clinically significant sleep problems. Like most health problems, insomnia correlates with lower rather than higher socioeconomic status.

While common, **sleep problems** are far from trivial. Insufficient sleep is a risk factor for traffic accidents and heart disease. It also diminishes cognitive function, leading to decreased efficiency and productivity in the workplace.

After insufficient sleep, the body will try to make up for both missed delta sleep and REM sleep at the expense of the lighter stages of sleep. This phenomenon, called **rebounding**, suggests that both these stages have important physiological functions. REM sleep rebound is often associated with intensification of dreaming or nightmares when people recoup sleep after a period of insomnia.

DSM-IV recognizes two categories of sleep disorders, the **dyssomnias** and the **parasomnias**. It also includes categories of sleep disorder due to other psychiatric conditions (e.g., depression, psychosis, alcohol abuse or dependence) and sleep disorder from medical conditions other than alcohol. Dyssomnias are, by definition, disorders of initiating or maintaining sleep. Parasomnias are abnormal sleep-related events (covered below). As an abnormal event occurring during sleep, somnambulism is a parasomnia.

The **treatment of mild sleep disorders** centers on adherence to a behavioral protocol that encourages sleep, called **sleep hygiene**. Good sleep hygiene involves eliminating barriers to restful sleep, including caffeine, tobacco and alcohol, over or undereating in the evening, exercising too late in the day, noise and extremes of temperature. All these measures reflect common sense. Behavioral research has contributed three other points of sleep hygiene: the importance of avoiding daytime naps, the helpfulness of a fixed rising time every morning (regardless of when the person goes to sleep), and advice not to stay in bed awake or involved in any nonsleep activity for any length of time.

The **fixed rising time** relates to the ease with which some people's sleep cycle creeps forward, because humans' biological clocks naturally run longer than 24 hours. Environmental regulators or *zeitgebers*, especially light, help keep circadian rhythms synchronized with the normal day/night cycle. Fixed rising functions as a *zeitgeber* to prevent phase advance.

The avoidance of **nonsleep activity** exemplifies applied conditioning. People who read, work, watch TV, or merely fret about not sleeping while lying in bed condition themselves to wakefulness there. Using the bed for sleep and only sleep, by contrast, conditions the person to drowsiness in the appropriate place.

Narcolepsy is a dyssomnia in which a person experiences irresistible sleep attacks at inappropriate times. These may be harmless, as when a person falls asleep during a monotonous sedentary activity, or harmful. Narcoleptics may fall asleep in the middle of conversations or, most alarming, while behind the wheel. Decreased REM latency characterizes the sleep EEG in narcolepsy. Patients immediately enter REM sleep, without the normal 90 minutes between falling asleep and the first REM period. Genetics accounts for a remarkably high percentage of this disorder; 90-100% of narcoleptic patients have the HLA-DR2 histocompatibility antigen, compared with 10-35% of the general population. The proportion of afflicted first degree relatives in patients with narcolepsy is up to 50% in some studies.

216

In addition to the characteristic sleep attacks, narcoleptic patients have associated symptoms of cataplexy (sudden paralysis of motor activity while awake), hypnagogic hallucinations, and sleep paralysis (inability to move while falling asleep). All presumably represent the inappropriate occurrence of parts of REM sleep. Of the associated findings, cataplexy is the most common, occurring in up to 80% of cases.

Of all the sleep disorders, **sleep apnea** probably has the greatest medical significance. Sleep apnea connotes the presence of five or more periods per hour or 30 or more periods a night of cessation of respiration for 10 seconds or longer. In central sleep apnea, the person makes no respiratory effort during these times; in obstructive sleep apnea, abdominal and thoracic muscle activity increases, but the person cannot move air past nasal-pharyngeal obstruction. Pure central sleep apnea accounts for only 10% of cases. Most sleep apnea is either obstructive or mixed. Each period of apnea terminates with momentary arousal, so that total sleep and sleep quality (decreased amounts of stage 3 and 4) both diminish.

During apnea, hypoxia, hypercarbia, and acidosis occur, predisposing the person to cardiac arrhythmias. Transient pulmonary and systemic hypertension (but not orthostatic hypotension) also occur and may become persistent in longstanding, severe cases. Behaviorally and symptomatically, apneic episodes are associated with snoring and snorting, sweating, sleepwalking, sleeptalking, and gastroesophageal reflux. Patients may awaken with headaches, possibly related to the dilation of cerebral blood vessels during the night. Obesity, once thought to cause sleep apnea, may in fact be a sequela, due to decreased metabolism from recurrent hypoxia. Sexual dysfunction is another associated finding. Hypothyroidism, sinus or nasal obstruction, and acromegaly all predispose to sleep apnea. Untreated sleep apnea increases mortality.

Deficient total sleep and poor sleep quality in patients with sleep apnea lead to daytime sleepiness, often severe enough to impair work performance and automobile safety. Personality changes (irritability and anxiety) also occur, along with mood disorders and significant psychosocial distress, especially marital and occupational problems. Compensatory abuse of alcohol (for anxiety) or stimulants (for sleepiness) can become problems in and of themselves.

Sleep apnea is more common in males than females (10:1), though the incidence in females rises after menopause. Incidence rises in both sexes with age; from 30-67% of elderly males are affected, leading to speculation that apnea contributes significantly to pulmonary and cardiovascular deaths in this group, especially during sleep.

The patient in Item 474 suffers from **delayed sleep phase disorder**. (Patients who fall asleep too early and waken too early have **advanced sleep phase disorder**). As described above, delayed sleep phase disorder may reflect the natural tendency of the human circadian cycle to run longer than twenty four hours, effectively pushing the hour of sleep later and later in the absence of a daily structure that forces the person to awaken early. College and professional students are particularly prone to this pattern.

Nocturnal myoclonus (periodic limb movement disorder) and **restless legs syndrome** are two dyssomnias that may be easily confused with one another. Myoclonus refers to twitching or kicking of the lower extremities during sleep, leading to momentary arousals which patients typically do not recall. They do not experience any unusual sensations while awake; the diagnosis is typically made upon the history given by a bed partner or by polysomnography. Restless legs syndrome (**Ekbom's syndrome**) is a sensory disorder. Patients experience a creeping feeling and will move, stretch, or pace to relieve the symptom. This leads to difficulty falling asleep.

Both conditions are mainly idiopathic. Myoclonus may be associated with hepatic or renal failure, narcolepsy, and sleep apnea. Restless legs syndrome has been found in association with vitamin B_{12} or iron deficiency, pregnancy, temperature extremes, leukemia, rheumatoid arthritis and fibromyalgia. Sedative, alcohol, or other drug withdrawal, renal failure, and tricyclic antidepressants may contribute to either disorder. Restless legs syndrome may also occur in patients taking dopamine blocking drugs (antipsychotics). In this context it may represent the extrapyramidal side-effect of akathisia (inability to remain in a fixed position). Either condition may interfere with the quality of sleep and with daytime functioning, though restless legs syndrome seems more often associated with mood disorders and psychosocial impairment.

Match the **MOST** appropriate treatment in the answers below with the vignettes in the items below. Answers may be used once, more than once, or not at all

(A)	Bright light in the early part of the day
(B)	Bright light in the later part of the day
(C)	Improved sleep hygiene (avoid stimulants and alcohol, establish an effective bedtime routine, increase afternoon exercise, no nonsleep activities in bed), relaxation exercises
(D)	Advise the patient to establish a fixed bedtime and stick to it
(E)	Advise the patient to establish a fixed rising time and stick to it
(F)	Advise the patient to stay awake two hours later each night until the onset of sleep advances to a normal bedtime, then stick to it
(G)	Advise the patient to go to bed one hour earlier each night until reaching a normal bedtime, then stick to it
(H)	Continuous positive airway pressure, possible surgery
(I)	Occasional use of a sedative hypnotic
(J)	Daily use of methylphenidate or another stimulant
(K)	Prescription of nontricyclic antidepressant
(L)	Prescription of any antidepressant
(M)	Clonazepam, triazolam, levodopa/dopadecarboxylase, baclofen, or gabapentin
(N)	Referral to AA

476. Overweight 64-year-old man whose wife reports that he snores so loudly she has taken to sleeping in the spare room. He sweats profusely at night and complains of heartburn. Most mornings he wakens unrefreshed, with a headache. His blood pressure is typically 160/100. He takes several unrefreshing naps every day, even though this interferes with his work productivity.

477. A 24-year-old graduate student who falls asleep during lectures, so often that she must get other students' notes for most courses. She awakens from her naps feeling refreshed. Intense emotion causes her to abruptly lose muscle tone and collapse, without loss of consciousness. Some nights she experiences vivid hallucinations just as she is falling asleep.

478. A 45-year-old woman consults a psychiatrist for increased irritability and depression. She says she can't fall asleep at night because of needing to get up and move around to "work out the kinks" in her legs. She has taken to drinking two glasses of wine at bedtime--this puts her to sleep, but she wakes up several hours too early and can't get back to sleep until just before she needs to get up to go to work.

479.   A 65-year-old woman who complains that she can barely stay awake past 8:30 most nights. Because of this, she rarely goes out or sees friends in the evening. She awakens refreshed after a normal amount of sleep. In general she feels and functions well, but curtailing her evening activity contributes to chronic feelings of loneliness and isolation.

480.   A 20-year-old college sophomore cannot get himself to bed until well after midnight. Once he gets into bed, he falls asleep easily. He says he was "never a morning person," but he was able to get through high school using alarm clocks and relying on his mother to wake him in time. However, he now sleeps through two alarms. He would like to go to medical school but is unable to schedule morning classes or labs because he so often oversleeps.

481.   A 40-year-old man who complains of difficulty falling asleep for years. The problem started when he broke up with a girl friend of longstanding, but it has not resolved despite subsequent successful relationships. His sleep worsens when he is stressed, but he thinks part of the problem is that he worries so much about not sleeping, he can't relax enough to fall asleep.

482.   A 45-year-old woman with four month history of difficulty falling asleep and early morning awakening. She lies awake up to two hours at night and is up an hour before she needs to be, so that total sleep is diminished. She experiences daytime fatigue, low mood, crying spells, irregular eating, increased anxiety, and diminished self- esteem. No active medical problems.

ANSWERS AND TUTORIAL ON ITEMS 476-482

The answers are: **476-H; 477-J; 478-M; 479-B; 480-F; 481-C; 482-L**. Item 476 is a classic description of **sleep apnea**, which may sometimes be effectively treated with continuous positive airway pressure (CPAP). Definitive treatment of obstructive sleep apnea may involve surgery to correct whatever nasopharyngeal problem produces the obstruction. Central sleep apnea, which is rarer and can be reliably differentiated from obstructive sleep apnea only by polysomnography, is harder to treat. Though it may respond to CPAP, this treatment can also make it worse. Various drug treatments have been tried. The treatment of last resort is either diaphragmatic pacing or mechanical ventilation. Patients should avoid all sedative hypnotics. Concurrent depression may require antidepressant treatment with less sedating (mainly nontricyclic agents) and concurrent anxiety will sometimes improve with buspirone.

The patient in Item 477 has **narcolepsy**, manifested by sleep attacks from which she awakens refreshed, cataplexy and hypnagogic hallucinations. Efforts to ensure adequate nighttime sleep and prescribed naps may help, but stimulants like methylphenidate are specific remedies and the treatment of choice. Cataplexy responds to REM-suppressing agents like tricyclic antidepressants. Education and supportive psychotherapy may also be needed.

The patient in Item 478 illustrates **restless legs syndrome**, complicated by the inappropriate use of alcohol. Alcohol is a poor sedative because its short half-life ensures patients will enter into withdrawal in the middle of the night. If they awaken, return to sleep may be quite difficult. Treatments for restless legs syndrome (and for nocturnal myoclonus) include the long-acting benzodiazepine clonazepam or the short-acting triazolam (with drug holidays to minimize dependence), levodopa/dopa decarboxylase, baclofen and, most recently, gabapentin. When an antidepressant is also indicated, nontricyclic agents are preferred.

The patient in Item 479 illustrates **advanced sleep phase disorder**, which is more common in elderly people. Use of extremely bright light in the early evening may be effective in pushing back the onset of sleep to a more socially appropriate hour.

The patient in Item 480 illustrates **delayed sleep phase disorder**. When mild, this may respond to the advice to get out of bed at the same time each morning regardless of how long the patient has been asleep. However, patient 480 is unlikely to be able to follow such advice. Efforts to move the onset of sleep backwards in graduated steps always fail. Sleep phase advance, delaying the onset of sleep by two hours each day until reaching a normal bedtime, does work. This treatment requires strong motivation, since it forces the patient to miss four or five waking days and to stay up for several nights, disrupting social and occupational life to a severe degree. Once patients achieve a normal bedtime, they need to be very conscientious about sticking to it and to a fixed awakening time, or else their sleep will again naturally advance to its previous rhythm.

The patient in Item 481 has classic **psychophysiologic insomnia**, in which a period of insomnia related to a particular stress leads to conditioned anxiety about not being able to sleep and continued insomnia. Improved sleep hygiene, coupled with relaxation exercises (sometimes adding cognitive therapy to change the patient's negative expectations about sleep), is often effective. Because the condition is chronic, the use of sedatives is likely to be ineffective due to the development of tolerance and/or dependence.

The patient in Item 482 has a sleep disorder in the context of an episode of major **depression**. Successful treatment of the depression with any antidepressant will typically relieve the sleep disorder as well.

Items 483-490

Choose the **BEST** response.

483. All the following are considered parasomnias **EXCEPT**:

   (A)   nightmare disorder
   (B)   REM sleep behavior disorder
   (C)   sleep terror
   (D)   sleepwalking
   (E)   sleeptalking

484. Nightmare disorder differs from sleep terror disorder (*pavor nocturnus*) in

   (A)   clustering in the first third of the night
   (B)   being often associated with sleepwalking
   (C)   occurring mainly during REM sleep
   (D)   A and C only
   (E)   A, B, and C

485. Sleepwalking

   (A)   typically occurs during delta sleep, usually in the first third of the night
   (B)   occurs at least once in up to 15% of normal children
   (C)   tends to be familial; often outgrown in adolescence
   (D)   A and C only
   (E)   A, B, and C

486. All the following psychiatric disorders may be associated with complaints about sleep **EXCEPT**:

   (A)   schizophrenia
   (B)   depression
   (C)   antisocial personality disorder
   (D)   delirium
   (E)   anxiety disorders

487. During early sobriety, the sleep of alcoholics

   (A)   nearly always normalizes
   (B)   may be persistently extended or deepened
   (C)   may be fragmented, with diminished deep sleep
   (D)   is disrupted by sleepwalking
   (E)   None of the above

222

488. Which of the following polysomnographic findings are characteristic of a major depressive episode?

    (A)   shortened REM latency (early onset of REM sleep)
    (B)   increased REM density (increased frequency of eye movements) in the first half of the night
    (C)   decreased proportion and amount of delta (deep) sleep
    (D)   A and C only
    (E)   A, B, and C

489. Rebound insomnia may occur following the discontinuation of

    (A)   a sedative hypnotic
    (B)   a stimulant
    (C)   an antidepressant
    (D)   A and C only
    (E)   A, B, and C

490. Benzodiazepine sedative hypnotics should be prescribed for time-specified periods in the lowest effective dose

    (A)   to minimize dependence
    (B)   to lower the risk of suicide from overdose
    (C)   to minimize tolerance
    (D)   A and C only
    (E)   A, B, and C

ANSWERS AND TUTORIAL ON ITEMS 483-490

The answers are: **483-E; 484-C; 485-E; 486-C; 487-C; 488-E; 489-D; 490-D**. The **parasomnias** are abnormal sleep-related events. They include all the terms on the list except sleeptalking. Although abnormal, talking during sleep is not dangerous and does not impair function, so it is not a disorder. The other parasomnias are sleep bruxism (tooth grinding) and REM sleep behavior disorder, in which patients can injure themselves or bed partners enacting dreams.

Pavor nocturnus, or night terrors or sleep terror, is a dramatic disorder in which patients partially awaken screaming from stage four (deep) sleep. Patients are difficult to arouse. They can give no reason for the terror and are often amnestic afterwards. The disorder is most common in prepubertal children. Because it occurs during stage 4 sleep, it is most common in the first third of the night and is associated with another parasomnia of stage 4, sleepwalking. Nightmares, by contrast, are typically REM-related. Patients awaken to full alertness with memories of dream content. This disorder clusters in the second half of the night, when REM sleep predominates.

Many psychiatric disorders, including psychoses, delirium, dementia, depression, mania, substance use, and anxiety disorders, have prominent symptoms of **disturbed sleep**. When the sleep problems are severe enough to require clinical attention, they may be separately diagnosed as "insomnia or hypersomnia secondary to another Axis I or Axis II disorder". Antisocial personality disorder does not entail sleep problems.

During the acute drinking and early sobriety phases of their illness, **alcoholics** have many sleep problems. Active drinking can produce hypersomnia and difficulty awakening and/or insomnia in the second half of the night. Early sobriety is associated with marked insomnia and fragmentation of sleep. This can persist for weeks and may be sufficiently severe to precipitate a return to alcohol use.

The sleep disturbances of **depressed patients** have been well studied and include all the findings listed. When effective, antidepressants tend to normalize the sleep EEG, prolonging REM latency, decreasing REM intensity and making sleep more restful.

Rebound insomnia may occur from the withdrawal of any drug that affects sleep, especially the sedative hypnotics and the antidepressants. During rebound, patients experience difficulty falling and staying asleep and increases in REM sleep, associated with intense dreaming and awakenings. Stimulant withdrawal is associated with rebound hypersomnia, not insomnia.

The available **sedative hypnotics** all have some potential for abuse and dependence. This risk rises with persistent daily use. It may be diminished either by using the drugs for short periods (less than a month) or by using them only a few days each week. However, the great advantage of these drugs over older, barbiturate sedatives is that overdoses are rarely lethal unless they are combined with other drugs or alcohol.

CHAPTER XI
PSYCHOTHERAPY AND ETHICS

Items 491-502

Choose the **BEST** response.

491. Choose the **BEST** overall definition of psychotherapy.

    (A)   A method of treatment based on identifying the connections between early experience and current symptoms through interpreting patterns of thought that emerge when the mind wanders freely.

    (B)   A collection of specific, nonpharmacologic techniques for treating specific nonpsychotic psychiatric disorders.

    (C)   A healing relationship in which a therapist uses language and other symbolic human capacities to relieve patients' subjective distress.

    (D)   A method of relieving subjective distress through identifying and correcting distortions in patients' ideas about themselves and others.

492. Identify the **TRUE** statement(s).

    (A)   In meta-analyses of psychotherapy outcome, roughly 80% of patients show improvement, a number significantly greater than untreated controls.

    (B)   The degree of improvement is roughly equal across all forms of psychotherapy.

    (C)   In cost-effectiveness studies, psychotherapy substantially reduces the amount of money spent on general medical care.

    (D)   A and C only

    (E)   A, B, and C

493. All effective psychotherapies

    (A)   mobilize patients' hope for improvement

    (B)   involve interpretations that connect present and past, conscious and unconscious elements of patients' experience

    (C)   increase patients' sense of mastery

    (D)   A and C only

    (E)   A, B, and C

494. The **BEST** predictor of good psychotherapeutic outcome seems to be

    (A) the rigor with which the therapist adheres to a particular technique
    (B) the severity of the patients' presenting symptoms
    (C) the quality of the alliance between the therapist and the patient
    (D) the therapist's flexibility in using techniques from different types of psychotherapy, matching them to the patient's needs
    (E) the length of the therapy

Items 479-486

Match the kind of therapy in the answers below with the descriptive statements that **BEST** apply to them in the items. Answers may be used once, more than once, or not at all

    (A) Cognitive therapy
    (B) Psychoanalysis
    (C) Brief interpersonal therapy
    (D) Group psychotherapy
    (E) Individual psychotherapy
    (F) Rational emotive therapy
    (G) Past life therapy
    (H) Structural family therapy
    (I) Behavior therapy
    (J) Psychodrama
    (K) Narrative therapy

495. Enhances therapeutic efficacy through mobilization of universality, altruism, and cohesion.

496. Time-limited treatment approach that helps depressed patients recover from losses, role transitions, role disputes, or developmental deficits.

497. Addresses constellations of relationships (triangles, overclose bonds, or disengagement) that contribute to a range of individual problems including depression, disruptive behavior, and relapses of chronic illness.

498. An individual or group treatment designed to identify and correct conscious distorted or maladaptive patterns of thinking, especially those associated with depression and anxiety.

499. Enhances therapeutic efficacy by convincing anxious patients, especially those with phobias and panic, to expose themselves to circumstances that they fear.

500. General theory of human mental life and therapeutic change from which most other western psychotherapies derive, at least in part.

501. Therapy in which patients' early past experiences are thought to determine their perceptions of others, including the therapist, who focuses on identifying these patterns of thinking and relating to help patients develop greater self-awareness and improve their relationships.

502. Promotes improvement mainly through skill acquisition and desensitization.

ANSWERS AND TUTORIAL ON ITEMS 491-502

The answers are: **491-C; 492-E; 493-D; 494-C; 495-D; 496-C; 497-H; 498-A; 499-I; 500-B; 501-B; 502-I**. The term **psychotherapy** covers many different treatments, each with its own explanatory theory of conditions it purports to treat and of its own healing elements. The proliferation of theories and techniques obscures the core common threads that unite all psychotherapies. At the most general level, psychotherapy is a helping relationship in which a person shares his/her unique experience of self and world with a person specially trained to organize such information into a coherent conceptual framework that leads to changes in the sufferer's understanding and behavior. Different therapies do not treat specific syndromes the way that different antibiotics treat specific infections, though some make such claims. People need not have a diagnosable psychiatric disorder to respond to psychotherapy. With the possible exception of some anxiety disorders, moreover, disorders that respond to one psychotherapy are likely to respond to many others. Thus, answer B is incorrect. Answer A describes psychoanalytic psychotherapy and answer D pertains to cognitive therapy. While both are correct, neither serves as a definition of psychotherapy generally.

The evidence supporting the nonspecific nature of psychotherapy's effects comes from meta-analyses that show the "equal outcomes phenomenon." Comparisons between two forms of psychotherapy (e.g., cognitive vs. interpersonal therapy; individual vs. group; brief vs. open ended) support the finding that widely different therapeutic methods have similar effects. Sixty to eighty percent of patients improve following psychotherapy, regardless both of their presenting condition and of which form of treatment they undergo. It is important to note, however, that any therapy produces better outcome than no treatment. Psychotherapy is nonspecific, but not ineffective. The finding that the cost of providing medical care to distressed high users of services drops significantly when such people undergo psychotherapy illustrates that therapy is both efficacious and cost-effective.

Recognizing that all psychotherapies are effective has turned research attention to understanding the shared elements of all therapies. In addition to mobilizing hope and increasing patients' sense of mastery, all effective therapies involve an alliance between sufferer and healer. Another shared element of effective therapies seems to be the controlled arousal of strong emotion, which may be necessary for shaking up patients' habitual ways of looking at things and opening their minds to alternatives. Interpretation as defined in answer B is a technique that may contribute to the efficacy of psychoanalytic therapies particularly, but is not an essential element of all therapies.

Various subclassifications of psychotherapy exist. Meaningful distinctions are those between individual, group, and family/couples psychotherapy, between psychodynamic, interpersonal, and cognitive psychotherapy, and between brief, time-limited, and open ended psychotherapies. Different categories of therapy appear to achieve the overall equal outcome by different means. Thus, group psychotherapy, which may be psychoanalytic, cognitive, psychodramatic or of many other derivations, has the power to reach people through unique elements common to groups. These include identification with other members (universality), helping other members (altruism), and closeness/acceptance within the group (cohesion).

Interpersonal psychotherapy was designed as part of a multisite research study comparing antidepressants and two different psychotherapies for the treatment of depression. Being constructed from clinical experience and from the epidemiological literature on depression, the therapy addresses specific circumstances thought to contribute to depression, including losses, transitions from one social role to another, conflict or detachment in important relationships (role disputes), and inability to make satisfying relationships (developmental deficits). Interpersonal therapy is focussed and time-limited. As one of few therapies studied with great rigor and proven successful in comparison to medication, many payers support it in some form. Thus, it is one of the more commonly available treatments in the current marketplace.

Structural family therapy is a form of treatment developed for helping families in which a child shows psychiatric symptoms, behavior problems, or unstable chronic illness. The theory behind it states that all symptoms and behaviors are forms of family communication. When the parental alliance is weak and parents are overly involved with one or another child (skew), or communicate through a child (triangles), the child becomes overwhelmed and develops psychological, behavioral, or medical symptoms. Treatment involves re-establishing appropriate boundaries between generations, realigning members so that people who were distant draw closer and those who were "enmeshed" achieve greater separation, and improving direct communication among family members to render communication through symptoms unnecessary.

Cognitive psychotherapy is a theory and method that repudiates the psychoanalytic tenet that the causes of psychological and behavioral symptoms must be sought in unconscious mental life, especially in conflicts between conscious beliefs and unconscious drives, fantasies, memories, and so on. Cognitive therapists focus on patients' consciously held beliefs about themselves, others, and the world in which they live. They identify characteristic distortions in the thinking of depressed and anxious patients and systematically teach patients to correct these distortions. Cognitive therapy is also called cognitive behavioral therapy, acknowledging elements borrowed from strict behaviorists. These include prescribing structured activities outside of therapy and encouraging the practice of new ideas in daily life. Cognitive therapy, like interpersonal psychotherapy, has been rigorously tested against medication and found to be effective for mild and moderate depressions. In the treatment of panic and phobias, it seems at least as effective as behavior therapy. Like all effective therapies for anxiety, cognitive therapy involves the element of exposure, of getting patients to confront what they have feared and avoided, until they achieve mastery of their reactions.

Strict behavior therapy derives from animal research and discounts the importance of human's perhaps uniquely evolved capacities for thought. Rather, the core element of this therapy is teaching people to behave in more adaptive ways, expecting their interpretation of experience to shift in consequence. The overlooking of symbolic thought is more apparent than real, since it takes considerable persuasion to get people to institute the recommended changes in behavior. Behaviorists highlight the therapeutic role of skill acquisition and **desensitization**. An example of skill acquisition would be teaching alcoholics with intense social inhibition to relate to others while sober. Desensitization involves exposing patients to previously feared or avoided situations until they no longer react to them. This can be done gradually, advancing patients by degrees toward a feared circumstance and teaching or allowing them to become comfortable at each step. Flooding, another form of desensitization, involves having a patient endure a feared situation and the distress it brings at great intensity until the distress subsides. Flooding teaches the person that he or she can withstand these feelings and that they will end. Either method of desensitization seems to be a core element of all psychotherapies that relieve anxiety. This is the one instance in which the universal outcomes phenomenon may not apply. Therapies that omit exposure do not work as well for anxiety as therapies, either behavioral or cognitive behavioral, that include this element.

Psychoanalysis, a theory of human mental life and of psychological symptom formation, is the forerunner of all contemporary psychotherapies, either directly or because other therapies were developed to challenge it. As a theory which evolved over a span of five decades, psychoanalysis has many different facets, not all of which are internally consistent. Certain features, however, are characteristic. These include the postulate that adult beliefs about the self and others and patterns of relating are determined by experience with important other people earlier in life, and that therapeutic change requires making these early experiences conscious and their influence explicit. Analysts identify the effects of patients' earlier experience by their effect on the person's relationship to the therapist. Patients are thought to transfer beliefs, emotions, and patterns of interaction from their earlier relationships into therapy. Interpretation of this **transference**, making the links between past and present explicit, is considered a core element of psychoanalytic treatment, regardless of the presenting symptom.

Items 503-512

After each vignette in the items below, chose the **MOST** appropriate form of psychotherapy or the **BEST** response.

A 75-year-old woman whose husband died four years ago still has disturbed sleep, partial loss of pleasure and interest, crying spells and trouble maintaining her weight. She complains of multiple aches and pains and constipation and worries that the breast cancer she had treated at age 60 may be recurring. She denies alcohol or drug use and says that although she would welcome death, she would never try to hurt herself.

503.   The **MOST** appropriate form of psychotherapy would be

(A)   psychoanalytic psychotherapy
(B)   behavior therapy
(C)   brief interpersonal therapy
(D)   Emotions Anonymous
(E)   rational emotive therapy

504.   Useful adjuncts to her psychotherapy could include

(A)   widows' support group
(B)   Reach for Recovery
(C)   antidepressant medication
(D)   A and C only
(E)   A, B, and C

A 24-year-old graduate student experiences disabling anxiety symptoms when he must speak in class or in front of group. The patient also describes anxiety in informal social interactions. He rarely goes to parties or places where he might have to enter into conversations with strangers. He says he "feels stupid" and thinks others are irritated by his difficulty making conversation. His grades are suffering because of his inhibitions, and he is considering giving up his program to find a less stressful kind of job.

505.   The **MOST** appropriate form of psychotherapy would be

(A)   Emotions Anonymous
(B)   psychoanalytic psychotherapy
(C)   network therapy
(D)   cognitive behavioral therapy
(E)   vocational counselling

506.   His treatment might also include

    (A)   sertraline
    (B)   MAOIs
    (C)   propranolol
    (D)   A and C only
    (E)   Any of the above

A 35-year-old, divorced man gives a history of moderately heavy drinking for ten years. In the two years since his divorce he has been more depressed, with disrupted sleep, irritability, fatigue and cynicism. He admits that he typically drinks more than he intends to. On weekends, he can consume a case of beer in two days. Recently, he has begun drinking in the morning before work to relieve a persistent hangover.

507.   The **MOST** appropriate form of psychotherapy would be

    (A)   cognitive behavioral therapy
    (B)   self-help (AA or Rational Recovery)
    (C)   structural family therapy
    (D)   psychoanalytic psychotherapy
    (E)   interpersonal psychotherapy

508.   Prior to referral, this physician should

    (A)   initiate treatment with an antidepressant
    (B)   initiate treatment with disulfiram
    (C)   assess whether the patient recognizes that his drinking is dysfunctional and not fully under his control
    (D)   All of the above
    (E)   None of the above

A 25-year-old woman comes in confused and anxious about her relationships. She describes a pattern of being self-effacing in intimate relationships. She gets involved with men who initially seem charming and protective, only to find that they become dominating and verbally abusive as the relationship proceeds. Her current boyfriend has twice coerced her into sexual activity over her strong objections. The patient mentions that her parents' relationship was overtly abusive. After her parents divorced when she was 8, she lived with her mother, who did not remarry for ten years. During this time, the patient's mother had three or four boyfriends who were critical and demeaning, both of her mother and of her. At the same time, she discounts her feelings about this as "probably overreacting or something." She presents a cheerful, competent facade to the world but feels she "blocks out" a lot of her most painful feelings and memories as she has done at least since early adolescence.

509. The **MOST** appropriate form of psychotherapy would be

(A) psychoanalytically oriented psychotherapy, brief or long-term
(B) Emotions Anonymous
(C) assertiveness training
(D) Sex and Love Addicts Anonymous
(E) family therapy with her mother and stepfather

510. Treatment will likely also involve

(A) alprazolam
(B) valproic acid
(C) methylphenidate
(D) All of the above
(E) None of the above

A 12-year-old boy is repeatedly brought to the emergency room by his mother for episodes of asthma. His mother seems overwhelmed by the boy's condition; she complains that she can't get him to take his prophylactic inhalers regularly. Two younger children in the family are beginning to show behavior problems because their mother is so anxious and concerned about her oldest son. The patient's father never brings him in. He is described as kind but disengaged, working long hours and wanting only to be left alone when he comes home.

511. The **MOST** appropriate form of psychotherapy would be

(A) behavior therapy
(B) play therapy
(C) cognitive therapy
(D) family therapy with mother and son
(E) structural family therapy with both parents

Choose the **BEST** response.

512. Compared to professionally led groups, self-help programs are

(A) more effective
(B) more standardized and accountable
(C) cheaper and more accessible
(D) A and C only
(E) A, B, and C

ANSWERS AND TUTORIAL ON ITEMS 503-512

The answers are: **503-C; 504-D; 505-D; 506-E; 507-B; 508-C; 509-A; 510-E; 511-E; 512-C**. In Items 503 and 504, the patient's grief symptoms, though understandable, have persisted well beyond the usual two years of acute distress. She is now diagnosable as **depressed**. Interpersonal therapy for depression offers a protocol specifically for resolving depression after loss and is also compatible with antidepressant medication, which is indicated here. This patient might do as well in a widows' support group, if her depression is not so severe that it prevents her from attending. **Reach for Recovery** is a support program for women recovering from breast cancer surgery, not an appropriate resource in this phase of this patient's life. Her concern about cancer is a form of depressive somatic preoccupation and should not be the main focus of her current treatment.

In Items 505 and 506, the patient exemplifies **social phobia**. As an anxiety disorder with an element of panic, it may respond best to a treatment that involves **exposure** as a therapeutic component. Of the therapies on the list, cognitive behavioral therapy provides the best fit. **Emotions Anonymous**, a twelve step, self-help program for emotional dyscontrol, might work but only if the patient can calm his anxiety enough to actively participate and only if his world view is compatible with the program's emphasis on trusting a higher power. Emotions Anonymous is, moreover, a program that has never been professionally evaluated (unlike AA or Recovery, Inc.). A professional could not endorse it as strongly as **cognitive behavioral therapy**, which has a strong research base. Psychoanalytic psychotherapy, which characterizes social phobia as evidence of conflicts related to the Oedipal phase of development, might be effective, but only if modified to include some element of exposure, or if the patient spontaneously practices exposure in conjunction with the therapy. Network therapy is an intervention that prevents relapse in substance abusers. Vocational counselling is contraindicated. Suggesting it would only confirm this patient's view that his symptoms are severe, untreatable and permanently disabling.

Sertraline and **MAOIs** relieve autonomic symptoms and promote changes in the maladaptive beliefs of social phobia. Propranolol may help specifically with the element of tremor, if present, or of stage fright. However, it relieves only the peripheral autonomic symptoms. Except in performance anxiety, beta blockers are ineffective for the core manifestations of phobic disorders. Because this patient would still fear his reactions and the situations that provoke them, propranolol would be an adjunct to treatment, insufficient on its own. Some research suggests that bupropion, a dopaminergic antidepressant, might also be effective in social phobia, even though it is not effective in other anxiety disorders. Controlled studies of its efficacy in this condition, however, have not yet been done.

Items 507 and 508 pertain to a man with **alcohol abuse** proceeding to alcohol dependence. Individual psychotherapeutic approaches to this condition are generally ineffective. Group self-help, though not a panacea, is about as effective professional interventions for those who participate actively. The advantages of self-help compared to professionally led group programs are negligible cost, diversity of membership, flexibility, and constant/persistent availability. Its disadvantages include lack of accountability and the wide variation in quality among different groups ostensibly practicing the same method. Professional help may be needed to enhance patients' motivation to engage in self-help. Some patients who are alienated from self-help philosophies may benefit from professionally led groups. Patients with dual diagnoses also have problems participating in self-help groups focussed on substance abuse alone. Family therapy is a helpful component of treatment for alcohol abuse, but this patient does not have an intact family.

Alcoholics require at least one month of sobriety before they become candidates for **antidepressant treatment**. Many will find their depressive symptoms remit with abstinence alone. Thus, adjunctive antidepressant treatment is not indicated in this patient at the time of initial diagnosis, though it might be used later. **Disulfiram**, which precipitates a toxic reaction if patients drink alcohol, also cannot be used as an initial treatment, though it may help patients who achieve sobriety to maintain it. Professional assessment of the person's awareness of drinking as a problem is an important and necessary function. Recommendations for self-help only succeed in patients who have some inkling that they need it. Efforts to educate patients about the damaging effects of alcohol in general and about the role played by alcohol in their particular case contribute substantially to the success of treatment.

The patient in Items 509 and 510 would likely benefit from **psychoanalytically oriented psychotherapy**. Her complaints are more about self-concept, maladaptive defenses, and patterns of relationships than symptoms. The patient is aware, but only partially, that her earlier experience plays a contributory role. The nondirective stance of the psychoanalytic therapist would experientially encourage her to rely more on her own perceptions and judgment, by eliciting and relieving her discomfort in a situation where it is expected that she will experience distress. While therapy might lead or encourage her to become more assertive, assertiveness training per se does not address the many levels of her difficulty. Simple encouragement to be more assertive might even endanger her if her partner were to react with overt abuse or battering. Family therapy with her parents would have been more appropriate before she left home. It is no longer the current behavior of the family, but her internalized reactions to past experience, that shape her problem.

Symptomatically, this patient's misleading facade, vagueness and blocking out of painful affect and memory suggest the use of **dissociation** as a prominent psychological defense. No available medical treatments improve dissociation per se, so none are indicated here. Dissociation in the course of partial complex seizure disorders may improve with valproic acid. Methylphenidate improves focus in the context of attention-deficit/hyperactivity disorder. Alprazolam can sometimes relieve the anxiety that leads to dissociative reactions, but at the cost of exposing patients to the risks of addiction. Recognizing and changing maladaptive defenses like dissociation is a core element of psychoanalytic psychotherapy, so this aspect of her case may resolve with therapy alone.

The situation described in Item 511 exemplifies the family factors that may affect the stability of a chronic medical condition like asthma. Specifically, this patient's mother needs the support and involvement of another adult to help her modulate her anxiety about her son's illness. His natural push for independence, moreover, may be contributing to his opposition to using inhalers when she pushes him to do so. Involving his father in the struggle is likely to succeed because it rewards the son's desire for his father's attention and approval while defusing the intense, mutually frustrating interactions with his mother. Therapy with the mother and son alone, by contrast, tends to reinforce the existing maladaptive pattern of family relationships,

234

though it could work if the goal were to decrease rather than increase her involvement in his care. Play therapy is a form of psychoanalytic therapy adapted to the needs of younger children who have limited ability to express themselves verbally. Cognitive or behavioral approaches might work, but structural family therapy addresses the widest dimensions of the problem most directly.

Items 513-518

Choose the **BEST** response.

The patient is an 89-year-old, retired mathematician admitted to the hospital with pneumonia. In the course of diagnostic evaluation, his physician suspects lung cancer, which would require surgery and possibly chemotherapy. Upon hearing the news regarding his diagnosis, the patient becomes tearful and sad. He confides in his nurse his thoughts of suicide. The nurse also notices that the patient seems confused at times, not knowing the place and people who surround him. When the surgeon asks the patient to sign the informed consent for scheduled thoracotomy, the patient vehemently refuses any and all treatments of his condition, stating he is going to die anyway.

513.   In considering a further course of action, the surgeon should

(A)   Respect the patient's decision to receive no further treatment of his lung cancer, since the patient is clearly competent to make decisions about his medical care.

(B)   Disregard the patient's stated wishes and proceed with surgery, since the patient demonstrates impaired judgment as evidenced by his suicidality.

(C)   Request psychiatric consultation, since only psychiatrists are capable of verifying decision-making capacity in depressed patients.

(D)   Evaluate the patient for the presence of depression and delirium, as both of these conditions may impair judgement and decision-making capacity.

(E)   Refuse to treat the patient due to patient's lack of cooperation and refer him to a colleague.

514.   The ethical principle guiding the process of obtaining informed consent in this case should be the

(A)   principle of benign paternalism
(B)   principle of autonomy
(C)   utilitarian principle
(D)   principle of justice
(E)   principle of beneficence

515. All of the following are necessary components of a patient's capacity to give informed consent **EXCEPT**:

    (A)   Understanding the reason for a proposed treatment.
    (B)   Understanding the nature of the treatment.
    (C)   Understanding the probable outcomes and side-effects of the proposed treatment.
    (D)   Awareness of alternative treatments and the outcome of no treatment.
    (E)   Absence of evidence of delusions or hallucinations on the mental status examination.

516. Upon evaluating the above-mentioned patient, the surgeon discovers the symptoms of major depression. The next step in the management of this patient would be

    (A)   Scheduling of surgery, as it is clear that patient's ability to make rational decisions about his health care is impaired by the presence of depression, thus allowing the treating physician to make medical decisions for the patient.
    (B)   Contact the patient's family to obtain surrogate decision makers, who will act in the patient's best interest.
    (C)   Treat the underlying depression and reassess the decision-making capacity later.
    (D)   Petition the court for emergency guardianship.
    (E)   None of the above.

517. After successful treatment of the patient's depression, the patient continues to refuse surgery and chemotherapy. He demonstrates good knowledge of his condition, the proposed interventions, side-effects and alternative treatments, as well as the ramifications of no treatment, which include his death. The treating physician is to

    (A)   Consider the patient's age in his decision to refuse treatment.
    (B)   Respect the patient's stated wishes.
    (C)   Consider the wishes and feelings of the patient's children.
    (D)   Consider the benefit to society of patient's continued existence.
    (E)   Consider the legal ramifications to his own practice of medicine.

518. While the issues of informed consent and decision-making capacity are pondered, the patient experiences cardiac arrest. The physician then should

    (A)   Treat this emergency according to his best judgment.
    (B)   Recall that the patient did not want any treatment and not initiate resuscitation procedures.
    (C)   Consult the family regarding further medical interventions.
    (D)   Consult the court regarding further medical interventions.
    (E)   Proceed with management according to his understanding of the patient's wishes.

ANSWERS AND TUTORIAL ON ITEMS 513-518

The answers are: **513-D; 514-B; 515-E; 516-C; 517-B; 518-A**. When considering a patient's right to refuse or ability to consent to treatment, several issues must be addressed. One needs to consider the **competence**, or the decision-making capacity, of the patient in question. Other considerations include the **emergent nature of the condition, informed consent**, and the **ethical principles** guiding current practice of medicine.

First, in assessing a patient's refusal of treatment, the physician must ascertain whether the patient is capable, both mentally and psychologically, of making that decision.

Conditions that are known to temporarily or permanently cloud a person's ability to make decisions must be evaluated and treated, with the emphasis being on restoration of the patient's competence. The factors necessary to consider in competency evaluations are the patient's understanding of the nature of his or her illness and the proposed treatment, the side-effects of the treatment, the availability of alternative treatments, and the ramifications of no treatment. A decision based on a thorough understanding of these issues is referred to as informed consent. Pervasive depressed mood, clouding of consciousness, states of intoxication and withdrawal from drugs and alcohol all may affect a patient's capacity to make decisions. Therefore, conditions that can be treated or reversed must be eliminated prior to obtaining informed consent. In the case of the 89-year-old mathematician, suicidal thinking may point toward the diagnosis of depression, and confusion might indicate delirium. Both conditions have to be treated prior to further assessment of his decision-making capacity.

The ethical principle guiding the current practice of medicine is based on **autonomy theory**. Based on the writings of **Immanuel Kant**, autonomy theory postulates that the relationship between the physician and the patient is that of two responsible parties. This presumes responsibilities and obligations on the part of both people. Thus, a normal adult patient is deemed capable of making responsible decisions concerning his or her life and health, even if the decisions contradict the physician's recommendations based on consideration of the patient's best interest.

Paternalism can be defined as performing actions for others' benefit without requiring their consent. Paternalism in medicine is currently an acceptable practice only if the patient is incapable of making decisions due to mental illness, psychological distress or cognitive impairment. In that case, the physician is obligated to seek other sources who would be familiar with the patient's belief system and be able to tell what the patient would have wanted if he or she were able to make decisions. Only in cases of life-threatening emergencies, unavailability of family members, or uncertainty on the part of the doctor about the motivations of family members, is the physician allowed to make decisions for the patient, keeping in mind the patient's best interests.

The **utilitarian principle** demands maximizing the benefit to the greatest number of people in making decisions. It operates in medicine in the mandatory reporting of a number of communicable diseases and in quarantines.

When an adult is deemed **competent to make medical decisions**, no other considerations, such as age, family wishes, or benefit to society, are relevant in his or her refusing or consenting to treatment. If the physician perceives that actions requested by a patient contradict the physician's own ethical code, the physician has the right to refer the patient to someone who would feel comfortable providing services in accordance with the wishes of the patient. This is commonly the case in requests for elective abortion.

Items 519-521

Choose the **BEST** response.

Jeremy is a 29-year-old man who is seeking psychiatric consultation because of bouts of severe depression, accompanied by suicidal thoughts. Although well-educated, he is unable to get a job that fits his training, due to his illegal status in this country. He has been doing odd jobs, and barely makes a living. Additionally, his relationship with his girlfriend has become stormy over the last few months.

519. As Jeremy's physician and a responsible citizen, you must

    (A)   Report Jeremy's illegal status to the immigration authorities.
    (B)   Evaluate Jeremy's depression and assure his safety, especially in view of reported suicidality.
    (C)   Treat Jeremy's depression, refer him to a social service agency, and inform the immigration authorities of his illegal status.
    (D)   Consult your attorney as to your rights and responsibilities.
    (E)   Recommend that Jeremy return to his country of origin and pursue legal entry into the US.

520. In the course of your evaluation, Jeremy implores you to keep what he has to tell you confidential. You assure him that this constitutes your standard practice. Having been thus reassured, he tells you that his girlfriend has been giving him much trouble lately. During their fights, she has threatened to report Jeremy to immigration authorities. In response to this threat, Jeremy is planning to kill her. He has an elaborate plan and means to execute it. Your next step would be

    (A)   Continue to find out more about his plans to kill the girlfriend.
    (B)   Find out his girlfriend's location, address and telephone number.
    (C)   Do nothing; having promised Jeremy confidentiality, your hands are tied.
    (D)   Notify the police of Jeremy's stated intent.
    (E)   B and D only

521. You believe Jeremy's intent to kill his menacing girlfriend to be serious and suspect that the underlying cause of his fury and homicidality is his untreated depression. Your recommendation to him is to admit himself to a psychiatric hospital for further evaluation, treatment, and safety. He vehemently refuses. Under these circumstances, you can

   (A)   Having thoroughly explained to Jeremy the risks and benefits involved in his decision, and having deemed him to be a competent adult, leave the decision regarding hospitalization up to him.
   (B)   Call the girlfriend and other friends and relatives in the hope of influencing Jeremy to change his mind and consent to hospitalization.
   (C)   Proceed with the procedure for involuntary hospitalization.
   (D)   Call the police to have Jeremy arrested.
   (E)   Call a responsible adult who can assure the safety of Jeremy and his girlfriend.

ANSWERS AND TUTORIAL ON ITEMS 519-521

The answers are: **519-B; 520-E; 521-C**. The relationship between the physician and the patient is protected by the concept of confidentiality or **privileged information**. No information shared with the physician may be released to another party without the explicit and written consent of the patient. This includes release of medical information to other physicians and health care facilities. The right of the patient to confidentiality is protected by law. It is not only illegal, but unethical to notify the authorities of Jeremy's illegal status. The doctor's sole task in this case is to evaluate and treat Jeremy. The **exception to this rule** concerns information released to the physician that may threaten the life of the patient or others. Under these circumstances, the physician is not only allowed, but required to assure safety of the patient in the case of suicidal plans, and to notify the victim and the police in the case of homicidal plan. This is generally known as the **Tarasoff rule**, named after a case in California in 1976 where a therapist was found guilty for failure to inform the victim of a planned homicide. The physician has the responsibility to proceed with emergency detention of a clearly dangerous patient. In the presence of mental illness, the patient is to be detained in the hospital with the intention of providing treatment for the condition that led to the threat to self or others. If the patient refuses to admit himself to the hospital, the physician, in most states, is given jurisdiction to hospitalize the patient against his will for forty-eight hours. This allows the judicial process to be initiated, so that further treatment can take place.

INDEX

DSM, 49,51
DSM-IV, 52, 108
    , Axes I-V, 52
dyssomnia, 215

E-G

ego, 24
emotion, expressed, 68
encephalopathy, Wernicke's, 8
enlargement, ventricular, in autism, 76
ergotamine, 7
Erikson, Erik, 25, 26
examination, mental status, 58
Examination, Mini-Mental State (MMSE), 59
factors, risk for suicide, 65
fluoxetine, 125
fluphenazine, 125
forgetfulness, benign senescent, 97
Freud, Anna, 38, 42
    , Sigmund, 24, 38
functions, ego, 42
GABA, 21
galactorrhea, 16
gene, E4, 17
glycopyrrolate, 158
gyri, occipital, 12

H-K

haloperidol, 124
Harlow, Harry 25
Hartmann, Heinz, 42
5-HIAA, 66,143
history, family psychiatric, 54
hypnosis, 196
hypochondriasis, 192
hypomania, 208
hypotension, postural, 124
humor, 38
id, 24
idealization, primitive, 38
ideas of reference, 109
identification, projective, 38
impairment, neurological, 58

imprinting, 24
information, privileged, 239
inhibitors, serotonin-specific reuptake (SSRI), 20
insomnia, 216, 221
        , rebound, 224
intellectualization, 38
interview, psychiatric, 53
intoxication, 168
isolation of affect, 38
Kant, Immanuel, 237
Kraepelin, Emil, 49, 109

L-N

limbic system, 2, 8
lithium, 125, 151
lobe, dominant parietal, 12
lobotomy, 12
Lorenz, Konrad, 24
lymphocyte, -T, CD4, in AIDS, 99
Mahler, Margaret, 30
malingering, 192
mania, 11, 12, 62, 112, 146
MAOI, 125, 151, 152
    , and anxiety, 184
memory, 8, 59
meperidine, 195
methohexital, 158
methylphenidate, 82, 125
model, learned helplessness, 43
molestation, sexual, 32
myoclonus, nocturnal, 217
narcolepsy, 216
nefazodone, 150, 151
neuroleptics, in AIDS, 104
            , atypical, 129
            , side-effects, 124
norepinephrine, 10, 15
nortriptyline, 125
nuclei, 15
nucleus, basalis of Meynert, 16, 93

O-R

olanzapine, 20, 131

pain, acute, 195

parasomnia, 223

Parsons, Talcott, 47

passive-aggression, 38

paternalism, 237

patient, narcissistic, 48

    , paranoid, 47

    , schizotypal, 47

pavor nocturnus, 223

personality, 43

    , avoidant, 205

    , borderline, 205

    , narcissistic, 208

phenelzine, 125

phobia, social, 180, 223

physostigmine, 16

Piaget, Jean, 25

pimoline, 82

pimozide, 79, 83

placebo, 196

Pneumocystis carinii, 100

projection, 38, 40

propaphol, 159

pseudodementia, 97

pseudoparkinsonism, 47

psychoanalysis, 229

psychosis, schizophreniform, 62

psychotherapy, 227

    , cognitive, 228

    , interpersonal, 228

    , psychoanalytic, 234

    , psychodynamic, 54

quotient, intelligence (IQ), 72

rage, 4

rationalization, 38

RDC, 51

Reach for Recovery, 233

reaction formation, 38

realm, social, 20

receptor, α-adrenergic, 19

    , D_2, 19, 124

    , D_4, 19

thioridazine, 125, 184
tic, 79
thought, concrete, 25
    , formal operational, 25
    , preoperational, 25
torsade de pointes, 151
Toxoplasma gondii, 100
tract, tuberoinfundibular, 16
traits, borderline personality, 48
trazodone, 126, 150, 151
tubocurarine, 158
tyramine, 125

U-Z

utilitarianism, 237
Vaillant, George, 38
venlafaxine, 151
virus, human immunodeficiency (HIV), 99
Wechsler Intelligence Scale, 12
withdrawal, alcohol, 170, 175
    , amphetamine, 170
    , cocaine, 175
    , opioid, 170
    , sedative, 170
zeitgeber, 216